PAIN MANAGEMENT

*Evidence-Based Tools
and Techniques for
Nursing Professionals*

Yvonne M. D'Arcy, MS, CRNP, CNS

Pain Management: Evidence-Based Tools and Techniques for Nursing Professionals by Yvonne M. D'Arcy, MS, CRNP, CNS is published by HCPro, Inc.

Copyright 2007 HCPro, Inc.

All rights reserved. Printed in the United States of America. 5 4 3 2 1

ISBN 978-1-57839-964-2

HCPro, Inc., provides information resources for the healthcare industry.

HCPro, Inc. is not affiliated in any way with The Joint Commission, which owns the JCAHO and Joint Commission trademarks.

Yvonne M. D'Arcy, MS, CRNP, CNS, Author
Rebecca Hendren, Managing Editor
Emily Sheahan, Group Publisher
Jean St. Pierre, Director of Operations
Darren Kelly, Production Coordinator
Genevieve d'Entremont, Copyeditor
Alison Forman, Proofreader
Shane Katz, Cover Designer
Michael Roberto, Layout Artist

Advice given is general. Readers should consult professional counsel for specific legal, ethical, or clinical questions.

Arrangements can be made for quantity discounts. For more information, contact:

HCPro, Inc.
P.O. Box 1168
Marblehead, MA 01945
Telephone: 800/650-6787 or 781/639-1872
Fax: 781/639-2982
E-mail: *customerservice@hcpro.com*

Visit HCPro at its World Wide Web sites: *www.hcpro.com* and *www.hcmarketplace.com*

Contents

Chapter 3: Pain assessment

Chapter 4: Pain assessment tools and scales

Chapter 5: Pain medications

Chapter 6: Non-pharmacologic pain management therapies

Chapter 7: Acute pain management

Chapter 8: Chronic pain management

Chapter 9: Difficult to treat pain conditions and specialty populations

Bibliography

Nursing education instructional guide

About the author

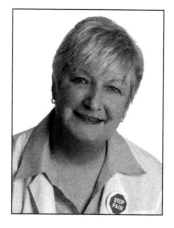

Yvonne M. D'Arcy MS, CRNP, CNS

Yvonne M. D'Arcy, MS, CRNP, CNS, is the Pain and Palliative Nurse Practitioner at Suburban Hospital in Bethesda, MD. She received her master's degree from Winona State University in 1995 as a clinical nurse specialist, and received her nurse practitioner certificate at the University of Florida in Gainesville in 1999. In addition, she pursued doctoral studies at the University of Florida and the University of Maryland in Baltimore.

D'Arcy has served on the board of directors for the American Society of Pain Management Nurses and served as chair of the Clinical Practice Committee of the American Society of Pain Management Nurses. She is a member of the International Association for the Study of Pain, American Pain Society, and the American Academy of Nurse Practitioners. In 2005, she was voted Advance Practice Nurse of the Year at Suburban Hospital and received the Lambert Foundation Award.

D'Arcy lectures and presents nationally and internationally on such topics as chronic pain, difficult to treat neuropathic pain syndromes, and all aspects of acute pain management. She writes frequently on various pain management topics and has been published in several prominent journals. In 2006, she received the Gold Award for best How to Series from the American Society of Healthcare Publications Editors for "A Fieldguide to Pain Management." She is currently on the editorial boards of *Nursing 2006*, *The Journal for Nurse Practitioners*, and *The Pain Medicine News*. She also participated in a review of the 2000 American Pain Society Arthritis Pain Guidelines and is one of the reviewers for the American Pain Society Low Back Guideline, which is currently in development.

Introduction

By Bill McCarberg, MD

Pain as a chief presenting complaint is the second most common reason for primary care visits. Pain accounts for one fourth of all sick time lost from work, or 50 million lost workdays per year (Brownlee and Schrof 1997). Almost 26 million people in the United States suffer from severe pain at least monthly. Despite the prevalence and enormous economic impact of pain, undertreatment is just as widespread. Fewer than half (43%) of Americans with moderate or severe pain feel that they "have a great deal of control" over their pain and 28% "don't believe that there is any real solution" for their pain (Pain in America 1997).

Our understanding about pain mechanisms and treatments is evolving faster than any other field of medicine. New drugs, drug combinations, and new uses of older drugs leave many providers wondering how to keep up with the knowledge. Reports appear almost daily of new discoveries about gene expression, drugs, infectious disease, the human genome, and pathophysiology. New interventional procedures require dedicated professionals just to keep up with the field.

This book is a comprehensive guide for nurses to help with pain assessment and treatment. The author is a nurse with broad experience in pain management and she is a leader in the field. Her background lends itself to the problems encountered by nurses in dealing with patients in pain. The information is practical and useful, and contains enough theoretical background to make the knowledge understandable.

Nurses have always had an advocacy relationship between physicians and patients. The constant exposure nurses have to patients during normal activities allows for observation of pain experiences that can be different than those patients describe to the physician. Patients rely on nursing staff for compassion, empathy, and judgment, as well as to interpret daily pain symptoms. After developing a relationship, patients often trust a nurse to put together the pieces of a complex medical condition.

Pain is complex and ever changing, and this book offers a wealth of information. *Pain Management: Evidence-Based Tools and Techniques for Nursing Professionals* will help us solve the tragedy of undertreated pain that most of us have seen in our precious patients.

Bill McCarberg, MD, is the founder and director of the Chronic Pain Management Program at Kaiser Permanente, in San Diego, CA, and a member of the University of California Medical faculty (voluntary). He is a member of the American Academy of Family Physicians, the American Academy of Pain Medicine, the American Pain Society, and the International Association for the Study of Pain. He has many years of experience in pain management and frequently presents and writes on various aspects of pain management.

References

Brownlee, S., and Schrof, J.M. (1997) "The Quality of Mercy: Effective pain treatments already exist. Why aren't doctors using them?" *U.S. News and World Report*, March 17, 1997.

Mayday Fund and TBC Research. (1997). Pain in America: A survery of American Attitudes Toward Pain. Available at *www.painfoundation.org/page.asp?file=library/painsurveys.htm.*

The problem of pain

Learning objectives

After reading this chapter, the participant should be able to

- describe the problems associated with pain management

- differentiate between acute, chronic or persistent pain, and malignant or cancer pain

- discuss the importance of using national guidelines for pain management in practice

The basic concepts of pain management are presented in this chapter. It also discusses the widespread nature of pain and how the different types of pain are defined. The last sections of the chapter review the use of national guidelines, position statements, and practice standards for pain management. Pain assessment and treatment options are discussed in later chapters.

The prevalence of pain

Pain has no boundaries and can affect anyone, no matter what age or gender. Pain infiltrates everyday living and can significantly reduce the quality of life for those who are suffering. Since pain is such a universal condition, knowing how to assess and manage pain is vital for all healthcare professionals. Knowing how to manage pain effectively and using evidence-based techniques will provide nurses with confidence when dealing with patients who are in pain.

With the increasing emphasis on using evidence to support nursing practice, there are many practices that have been examined and found to be lacking. Taking a hard look at "the way we always did things" may show that newer techniques are better. For example, pain medications for postoperative patients used to be given via the intramuscular (IM) route. Current practice guidelines (APS 2003) indicate that this route is not effective for pain relief, both because of the irregular absorption of pain medication and because scarring can occur at the site of injection. Today most patients who receive postoperative pain relief are given medication via the IV route. Nursing practice can evolve when evidence-based guidelines are used.

Pain as a healthcare problem

The problem of pain is significant. Pain is the most common reason that patients make appointments to see their physician (APS 1999), accounting for approximately 40 million physician visits annually (Pain Advocacy 2004). The estimated cost of pain, related to absenteeism and decreased productivity, is calculated to reach billions of dollars annually (Roper Starch Worldwide 2002). More than 73 million surgeries take place annually, with 75% of these patients experiencing pain after surgery (Apfelbaum 2003).

These statistics point to the need for adequate pain management for patients, and the U.S. Congress has designated 2000 to 2010 as the Decade of Pain Control and Research, yet pain is still being undertreated. Nurses are in a powerful position for affecting change in the pain management situation. Nurses are advocates for patient care, are becoming more educated about how to manage pain, and are working toward improving pain management for patients.

Definitions of pain

Pain is most commonly defined as "an unpleasant sensory and emotional experience associated with actual or potential tissue damage, or described in terms of such damage" (Mersky 1979 in APS 2003). This definition clearly describes the elements of the pain experience:

- The unpleasant sensation

- The emotional component

- The realization that pain can be present without tissue damage

A more patient-focused definition states that "pain is whatever the person experiencing it says is occurring whenever the experiencing person says it does" (McCaffery 1968). This definition highlights the subjective nature of pain, in addition to its focus on the patient.

There are several different ways to classify pain, the most common being acute pain, chronic—often now called persistent—pain, and malignant or cancer pain. Each of the three conditions has a slightly different set of criteria. Additionally, pain from nerve damage is a special type of pain that is chronic in nature but can also be present in patients with cancer.

Acute pain

Acute pain usually has a short duration and an identifiable cause, such as trauma, surgery, or injury (APS 2003, ASPMN 2002). It is a signal to the body that something is wrong, and the patient expects to get better from this type of pain. Patients who are experiencing acute pain may have increased vital signs, such as elevated blood pressure or pulse (ASPMN 2002). However, chronic pain patients who are experiencing acute pain may not have these physiologic changes. This variability means nurses should not rely solely on changes in vital signs to determine if pain is present.

If acute pain continues untreated or is undertreated, it may lead to the development of chronic pain conditions, such as complex regional pain syndrome (CRPS), that are difficult to treat (D'Arcy 2006). Today, the recommendation is to treat acute pain aggressively, to limit the effect on the individual and to minimize the potential for the development of a more difficult to treat chronic pain syndrome (Acute Pain Management 2005, D'Arcy 2006).

The following are important elements of acute pain:

- Short duration

- Patient expects to recover

- May have increases in vital signs, unless the patient has an underlying chronic pain condition

- Untreated or undertreated acute pain may lead to disabling chronic pain syndromes, such as CRPS

Chronic or persistent pain

Chronic or persistent pain, as opposed to acute pain, is pain that lasts beyond the normal healing period of three to six months (ASPMN 2002). Additionally, there may be no easily identifiable cause (Acute Pain Management 2005). A patient who develops chronic pain—such as low back pain from an injury, or a painful condition such as diabetic neuropathy—also may develop depression (D'Arcy 2006). Changes in vital signs may not be present, as the patient's body has learned to cope with the stress of continued pain. For a patient with chronic pain—no matter what the cause—the changes in lifestyle, decreased self-esteem, and financial burdens can exacerbate the pain and affect relationships.

The following are important elements of chronic pain:

- Pain that lasts beyond the normal healing period.

- Does not need tissue damage to exist. Physical damage may not be evident on x-rays or radiologic scans such as MRIs and CT scans.

- Depression is common.

- Vital sign changes may not be evident.

- Affects all areas of the patient's life.

Cancer or malignant pain

Patients who are diagnosed with cancer may fear the pain they experience is associated with disease progression (NCCN 2000, APS 2005). Cancer pain can be the result of tumor growth, metastases, or cancer-related therapies such as radiation or chemotherapy. Cancer pain can be both acute and chronic in nature. For 20–75% of adult cancer patients, pain is present at the time of diagnosis. For adult patients with advanced disease or end-stage disease, pain may be present in 23–100% of all cases. Sixty-two percent of pediatric patients have pain at diagnosis, while 62–90% have pain at the end of life (APS 2005).

This overwhelming incidence of pain with cancer should suggest aggressive pain management. However, evidence suggests that even pain from cancer is being undertreated (AHCPR 1994, APS 2005). The National Comprehensive Cancer Network (NCCN) states that cancer pain could be well controlled for most patients if adequate assessment and pain management techniques were employed (NCCN 2000).

Adequate treatment for pain is especially important for this group of patients. Cancer patients fear the cancer diagnosis the most and then fear the pain that may follow. Almost all cancer patients have heard about or seen someone die in pain from cancer. The idea that they may die the same way frightens them and makes the pain even worse. Providing cancer patients with effective pain management provides the best quality of life and means that the thing the patients fear most has been overcome.

The following are important elements of cancer-related pain:

- Cancer pain can be the result of tumor growth, metastases, or the result of cancer treatment

- At some time in the illness trajectory most cancer patients will experience pain

- For up to 90% of all cancer patients, adequate pain control could be provided with present pain management methods (AHCPR 1994)

- Cancer pain should be controlled aggressively to give the patient the best quality of life possible

- Cancer patients may have combinations of acute, persistent, or neuropathic pain

Neuropathic pain

Neuropathic pain is the result of nerve damage (Staats et al 2002) and can be from damage to the central nervous system, such as post stroke pain, or the peripheral nervous system, such as postherpetic neuropathy (PHN) (ASPMN 2002). Patients with neuropathic pain will often describe the pain as burning, tingling, pins and needles, painful numbness, or shooting.

There are several different causes of neuropathic pain:

- Neuropathy from diseases or injury such as diabetes, postherpetic neuralgia, or CRPS

- Neuropathic pain syndromes as result of nerve entrapment or surgical damage, post thoracotomy pain syndrome, post mastectomy pain syndrome, phantom limb pain, and post hysterectomy pain syndrome

- Treatment-related neuropathic pain, such as chemotherapy-related neuropathies that develop with the continued use of vinca alkaloid chemotherapeutic agents

- Centrally originating pain, such as post stroke pain or spinal injury pain found in quadriplegics or paraplegics

The one similarity with all these pain syndromes is the high degree of difficulty in managing pain. Neuropathic pain is a pain that becomes self-promoting and continues to provide pain stimulus; therefore, patients with neuropathic pain syndromes suffer continually. They may also develop conditions such as allodynia or hyperalgesia, making the syndrome much more difficult to treat.

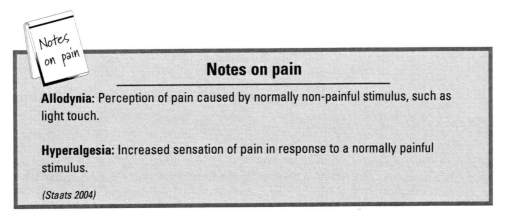

Notes on pain

Allodynia: Perception of pain caused by normally non-painful stimulus, such as light touch.

Hyperalgesia: Increased sensation of pain in response to a normally painful stimulus.

(Staats 2004)

Treating neuropathic pain requires the use of multiple medications, such as opioids, antidepressants, or antiseizure medications (Staats et al 2002). Since neuropthic pain is so difficult to treat, nurses should be supportive of patients with neuropathic pain syndromes, help them understand the pain, and educate patients about how to deal with these difficult-to-treat pain conditions.

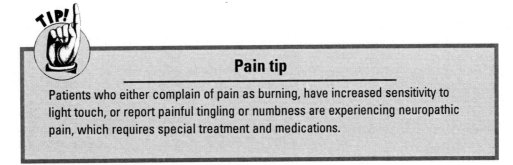

Pain tip

Patients who either complain of pain as burning, have increased sensitivity to light touch, or report painful tingling or numbness are experiencing neuropathic pain, which requires special treatment and medications.

National guidelines for pain management

Due to the widespread nature of pain and the damage it can do both physically, psychologically, and emotionally, efforts have been taken to help define the best practices for treating pain. The first efforts to set standards of practice for pain management were undertaken by the Agency for Health Care Policy and Research (AHCPR) in 1992. This body had panels of experts in the field develop pain guidelines for acute pain, cancer pain, and low back pain (AHCPR 1992, 1994).

As the work became too burdensome, the AHCPR turned over the process of guideline development in pain management to the American Pain Society (APS). This group continued to use panels of experts to develop guidelines for managing pain in specific settings and diseases. Some of the guidelines that have been developed include the following:

- Principles of Analgesic Use in the Treatment of Acute Pain and Cancer Pain, 5th ed. (2003)

- Guideline for the Management of Acute and Chronic Pain in Sickle-Cell Disease (1999)

- Guideline for the Management of Pain in Osteoarthritis, Rheumatoid Arthritis, and Juvenile Chronic Arthritis (2002)

- Guideline for the Management of Fibromyalgia Syndrome Pain in Adults and Children (2005)

- Guideline for the Management of Cancer Pain in Adults and Children (2005)

- Pain Control in the Primary Care Setting (2006)

- Low Back Pain Guidelines (in development; expected to be released in 2007)

- Opioid Use (in development)

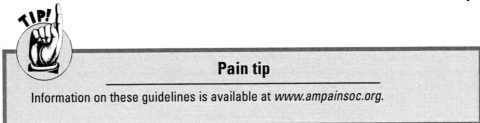

Pain tip

Information on these guidelines is available at *www.ampainsoc.org*.

In addition to the APS, many national specialty organizations have developed guidelines for pain management in their patient populations. For example, the American Geriatrics Society (elderly patients), the American Pediatric Society (infants and children), and the NCCN (cancer patients), all have disease-specific pain guidelines. Information on how to access these guidelines can be found in the practice exercises at the end of this chapter. One of the strongest national guidelines to date has been the standards developed by The Joint Commission (formerly known as the Joint Commission on Accreditation of Healthcare Organizations or JCAHO). These standards guide the practice of pain management in all hospitals that the regulatory body surveys, and hospitals must comply with the requirements of The Joint Commission Pain Management Standards to maintain accreditation.

Which recommendation should you use?

When determining how to use the recommendations for pain management in different populations and with different diseases, it is helpful to understand the strength of the different recommendations. Often the terms "standard," "consensus statement," or "guideline" are used interchangeably, but there are significant differences, as shown in the following definitions. When deciding on an intervention for pain management, use the one that has the highest level of support.

1. **Guidelines:** Systematically developed statements using an analysis of current research that can help practitioners make patient care decisions about appropriate healthcare for specific clinical circumstances (Berry et al 2003). Recommendations for practice are made using an evidence rating scale from poor support to high level support for treatment options. Examples of guidelines are the APS Pain Management Guidelines for sickle cell disease or arthritis.

2. **Standards:** Criteria established by authority or general consent as a rule for the measure of quality, value, or extent. Standards can be used to provide accreditation, and establish expectations on how pain should be managed in organizations. Examples of standards are those issued by The Joint Commission and by the Commission on Accreditation of Rehabilitation Facilities (CARF).

3. **Consensus statements and position papers:** Expression of opinion or positions—usually prepared by societies, organizations, or academies—to reflect the findings of the society. The formulation of these documents includes expert opinion, available scientific evidence, and prevailing opinion (Berry et al 2003). An example of a position statement includes the American Society of Pain Management Nurses (ASPMN) position statement on treating pain in patients with addictive disease.

The recommendations that have the strongest effect on pain management are standards, since they set out specific requirements that must be met for accreditation. Guidelines use a wide variety of resources and include a statement about the strength of evidence for recommendations for determining patient care. Position statements reflect the findings of a specific body of practitioners for a select indication. One important distinction to keep in mind is the difference between the legal use of standard of care (as determined by the practitioners in a specialty area) versus the standard using the criteria for accreditation.

Differences and similarities of standards, guidelines, and position statements

Similarities
1. Often multidisciplinary
2. Compliance is considered voluntary
3. Can be used to develop expected levels of performance
4. Can provide education for clinicians and the healthcare community at large

Differences
1. Standards are seen as authoritative, guidelines as recommendations
2. Audiences differ
3. The degree of clinical certainty can vary depending on the available scientific evidence

(Adapted from Berry et al 2003)

When to use a standard, guideline, or consensus statement is determined by the clinical needs of the patients. If the patient is in a hospital, The Joint Commission standard would be used. If a nurse wanted to know how to manage a specific type of pain, such as from sickle cell disease, a guideline would be the best option. Nurses working with patients who have an addictive disease would find the ASPMN position statement helpful.

The role of nursing in pain management

Nurses play a role in every aspect of pain management:

- Nurses are key to assessing pain

- Nurses have a holistic approach and determine what the overall effect of the pain is for that individual

- Nurses advocate for patients and expect that easing pain is a part of their professional responsibility

For nurses, seeing patients suffer is intolerable. Most nurses use every bit of knowledge and experience to help patients achieve an acceptable level of pain control. Perhaps more importantly, nurses continue to educate themselves about pain management and the latest techniques and medications. Using their special talents, nurses use non-pharmacologic methods for pain relief and try to empower patients to help control their pain.

Using evidence-based nursing to treat pain is important because it

- gives the nurse confidence in the intervention

- provides the most current information on medications and pain relief techniques

- can improve patient outcomes

- contributes to compliance with The Joint Commission requirements for pain management

- encourages high-quality nursing practice

(Adapted from Beyea & Slattery 2006)

Because nursing is such an integral part of successful pain management, it is critical that nurses take the time to look at the evidence for the various techniques and interventions. Using the methods that have the most research support allows the nurse to provide options for pain control that have the best chance for success. The following chapters present the latest research that can help all nurses better manage pain in their patients.

Case study: Mrs. Jones

Mrs. Jones, age 72, comes in to the emergency room complaining about ankle pain. She says she hurt her ankle when she tripped over the step to her house as she came back in from gardening. The ankle is red, swollen, and painful to the touch. She tells you the pain is sharp and rates it at 5/10 (moderate level pain) when she tries to walk and at 2–3/10 (mild pain) when she is resting. It hurts more when she tries to put her weight on it. She tried some over-the-counter medication for pain that helped only a little. She tells you she has had arthritis for many years and is almost always in pain.

Questions

1. What type of pain does Mrs. Jones have with her ankle?

Acute.

2. Do you think she has more than one type of pain?

Yes; she has chronic pain from the arthritis and acute pain from the injury.

3. Is there any indication that neuropathic pain is present? Does the patient have allodynia or hyperalgesia?

No.

4. Do you think Mrs. Jones will have elevated vital signs?

Mostly likely she will have some physiologic indication since she is having acute pain.

For the chronic arthritis pain her vital signs would not be a good indication of pain.

5. Is Mrs. Jones at risk for exacerbating her chronic pain condition if the pain continues?

Yes. If the pain continues to be undertreated or untreated, the patient is at risk of developing a more difficult to treat pain condition such as CRPS.

6. Since Mrs. Jones is elderly, do you think the pain should be treated conservatively or more aggressively?

The pain should be treated aggressively to avoid developing another chronic pain condition.

Practice exercises

1. Log on to the Cochrane Collaboration Web site at *www.cochrane.org* and search the database for pain management topics. Read some of the reviews, such as the one on low back pain. Was the information useful? Did you learn something you did not know about low back pain?

2. Search some of the organization Web sites listed below and determine what types of pain management information they provide. Which of the sites would be most useful in your practice?
   1. American Pain Society (APS): *www.ampainsoc.org*
   2. The American Academy of Pain Medicine (AAPM): *www.painmed.org*
   3. American Society of Addiction Medicine (ASAM): *www.asam.org*
   4. Pain and Policies Study Group at the University of Wisconsin Comprehensive Cancer Center: *www.painpolicy.wisc.edu*
   5. American Society for Pain Management Nursing: *www.aspmn.org*
   6. American Geriatric Society: *www.americangeriatrics.org*
   7. American Chronic Pain Association: *www.theacpa.org*
   8. American Pediatric Society/Society for Pediatric Research: *www.aps-spr.org*

The transmission of pain

Learning objectives

After reading this chapter, the participant should be able to

- define the four stages of pain transmission

The transmission of pain is a complex phenomenon that takes only milliseconds. Acute pain is meant to warn the body that an injury or damage has occurred. Persistent pain, because of its long-term nature, changes the way the body perceives and interprets pain. The information in this chapter will demonstrate the complexities of pain transmission and show how the body adapts to continued pain stimulus.

Ancient and modern theories of pain transmission

From the time of Renee Descartes, man has tried to determine how pain is transmitted (Arnstein 2002, Cervero 2005). The Descartes theory described the perception of pain as simply a stimulus-response phenomenon: the body is injured, so pain is experienced. Called the labeled line theory, it posits that a stimulus such as a burn travels from the affected area up to the brain, resulting in the recognition and sensation of pain. This in turn generates a response that travels back to the affected area and results in the appropriate behavior, such as moving the affected area away from the painful stimulus. Early efforts at discovering how pain is transmitted focused more on the physical transmission of pain, with little attention paid to the role of emotions and psychological responses.

See Figure 2.1 for a transmission of pain diagram.

Several pain theorists have suggested that pain has significant psychological and emotional components. As early as Aristotle, pain was identified as an emotional state (ASPMN 2002). However, not much is known about these facets. The fact that depression accompanies chronic or persistent pain is readily acknowledged, but whether the pain precedes the depression or follows it is still under debate (ASPMN 2002). Pavlov felt that pain was a learned response influenced by cultural and learned behaviors, and operant conditioning was the cure (Pavlov 1927, Fordyce 1976). In addition, others theorize that abnormal illness behaviors and pain behaviors are influential in the development of pain (Pilowsky & Spence 1976, Fordyce et al 1973).

Melzack and Wall, who formulated the Gate Control theory of pain in 1965, are perhaps the best-known pain theorists. Their theory explained that a pain stimulus can open a "gate" to transmit pain further up the nervous system.

The steps for pain transmission in the Gate Control theory are the following:

1. Continued painful stimulus on a peripheral neuron causes the "gate" to open by depolarization of the nerve fiber

2. Pain stimulus is then passed at a synaptic junction to the central nervous system

3. Pain stimulus passes up the central nervous system into the limbic system and cerebral cortex

4. Response to the pain is created in the cerebral cortex, and the response is then generated and passed to the efferent pathway, where the reaction to the pain is processed

This theory is still being updated and modified, with recent data indicating that the degree of the stimulus intensity can produce different responses. Additionally, pain-facilitating substances, such as Substance P, and pain-inhibiting substances, such as serotonin and opioids, can help open or block

FIGURE 2.1 **Transmission of pain diagram**

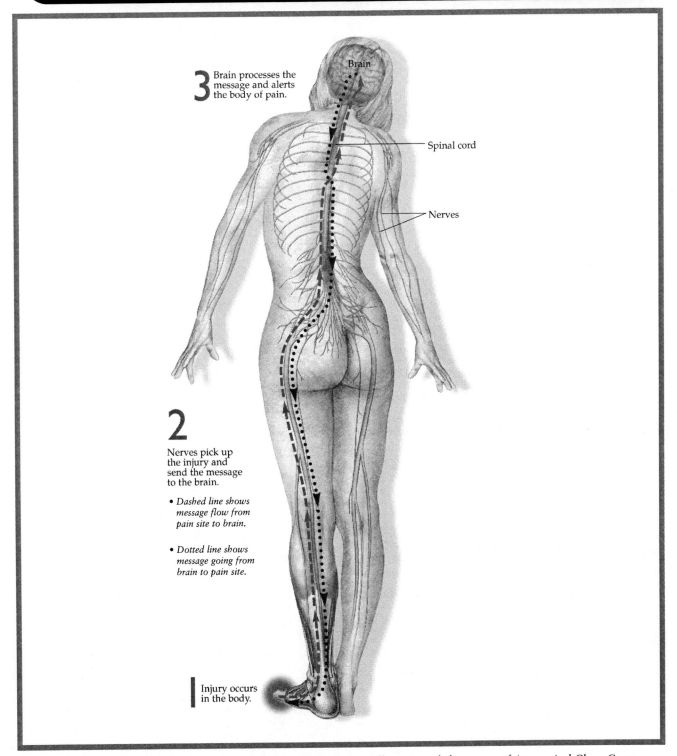

3 Brain processes the message and alerts the body of pain.

Brain

Spinal cord

Nerves

2

Nerves pick up the injury and send the message to the brain.

• *Dashed line shows message flow from pain site to brain.*

• *Dotted line shows message going from brain to pain site.*

Injury occurs in the body.

the action of the gate mechanism. Most of the recent research in this area centers on the way these substances create inhibition.

Another way of showing pain transmission is the *concept of nociception*, which is the perception of pain by sensory receptors called nociceptors. The four elements to this concept of pain transmission are transduction, transmission, perception, and modulation.

1. **Transduction:** Noxious stimuli convert energy into a nerve impulse, which is perceived by sensory receptors called nociceptors.

2. **Transmission:** The neural signal moves from the periphery to the spinal cord and brain.

3. **Perception:** The impulses transmitted to the higher areas of the brain are identified as pain.

4. **Modulation:** Inhibitory and facilitating input from the brain modulates or influences the sensory transmission at the level of the spinal cord (Berry et al 2006).

A pain stimulus is transmitted by two separate—but continuous—systems: the peripheral nervous system and the central nervous system. The pain stimulus, which leads to the sensation of pain as perceived by the patient, originates in the peripheral system and is relayed to the central nervous system on the afferent fibers.

Peripheral pain transmission

As pain is experienced, it is transmitted from free nerve endings in the periphery by A-delta nerve fibers and C nerve fibers. A-delta fibers are large nerve fibers covered with myelin that conduct pain impulses rapidly. C fibers are smaller and unmyelinated, and conduct pain impulses more slowly. The pain stimulus is transmitted by both types of nerve fibers from free nerve endings (nociceptors), resulting in the sensation called nociception (Edwards 2002).

> **Notes on pain**
> ---
> **Afferent nerve fibers:** Carry pain stimulus from the affected area to the central nervous system.
>
> **Efferent nerve fibers:** Carry the response away from the central nervous system to the affected area.

Nociception can originate in various locations:

- **Visceral:** Pain from visceral organs, often identified by patients as crampy or gnawing pain

- **Somatic:** Pain from skin, muscles, bone, and joints, often identified by patients as sharp pain

There are differences in the pain that is carried on the two different nerve fibers. A-delta fibers react quickly to a stimulus, and help the patient localize the origins of the pain. A pain transmitted on an A-delta fiber might be described as sharp or stabbing.

C fibers take longer to fire, and are responsible for the "achy" types of pain felt after the pain stimulus is removed. C fibers release Substance P, a neurotransmitter that is found throughout the nervous system where pain information is processed and helps to speed the transmission of painful stimuli along the pain pathway. Bradykinin is another pain-facilitating substance, found at injury sites as well as in the spinal cord pathways. Bradykinin acts as an irritant at the site of the injury and is similar to substance P.

Once a stimulus triggers a pain response at the free nerve endings, it travels along the peripheral nerve to the dorsal root ganglion, and from there, down the dorsal root into the posterior part of the spinal cord, known as the dorsal horn.

The following types of stimulus can trigger a pain response:

- **Mechanoreceptors:** action triggered by pressure

- **Thermal receptors:** triggered by heat or cold

- **Chemoreceptors:** triggered by certain chemicals, such as those found with inflammation

Central nervous system pain transmission

As the stimulus is delivered to the central nervous system via the dorsal root ganglion, it synapses in the substantia gelantinosa in the dorsal horn of the spinal cord and enters the central nervous system. Opening and closing the "gate" to nociception is controlled by the combined effect of both the summing up of the pain-facilitator impulses (substance P, bradykinin, glutamate) and the pain-blocking impulses (norepinephrine, serotonin, opioids) received in the substantia gelatinosa. Simplistically, if facilitator impulses predominate, the signal is sent on; if blocker impulses predominate, the signal stops. If the pain impulse is potentially life threatening, a reflex arc through the spinal cord will fire, causing immediate protective behavior (e.g., touching a hot stove leads to immediate withdrawal of the hand and arm). This can occur before any central nervous system processing of the pain stimuli (Cervero 2005).

Pain-facilitating and -blocking substances include the following:

- **Facilitating:** substance P, bradykinin, glutamate

- **Blocking:** serotonin, opioids, natural or synthetic, norepinephrine, GABA

From the dorsal horn in the spine, the pain crosses through the spinal cord into the lateral spinothalamic tracts, which lead directly to the thalamus, deep within the brain. From the thalamus, the signal goes into the limbic system, which controls the emotions associated with pain, and then to the cerebral cortex, where the stimulus is finally recognized as pain. This entire process happens within milliseconds.

The limbic system is thought to contain all the memories of previous painful events experienced by the patient. There are two neurotransmitters that are very important to pain transmission at this level: norepinephrine and serotonin. Some nerves use serotonin to produce firing impulses at synaptic junctions. Current therapies for chronic pain apply this concept by using tricyclic antidepressants (such as amitriptyline, desipramine, or nortriptyline) or selective serotonin reuptake inhibitors (such as fluoxetine or paroxetine) (APS 2003), which decrease serotonin available for release in the synaptic vesicles, thus decreasing the amount of neurotransmitter available to modulate the incoming pain stimulus. Glutamate is present in most fibers where it can be released to help facilitate pain transmission. It is the main neurotransmitter that is responsible for the communication of the peripheral nervous system with the central nervous system (Rowbotham, Kidd, and Porecca 2006). Additionally, glutamate is thought to play a role in the activation of N-methyl-D-aspartate (NMDA) receptors, which help prolong persistent pain (Merskey, Loeser, and Dubner 2005).

Once the pain stimulus is processed through the cerebral cortex, the descending nerve fibers from the locus ceruleus and periaqueductal gray matter transmit the response via the efferent pathway. In addition to norepinephrine and serotonin, other substances that can modulate the pain response at the dorsal horn are the naturally occurring opiates, endorphins and enkephalins. These substances are similar to morphine in their effects, binding opioid receptors in the dorsal horn of the spinal cord to block pain signal transmission. Aminobutryic acid (GABA) acts to inhibit pain transmission in the dorsal horn by acting on GABA-specific receptors (Scholz & Woolf 2006).

Response to pain stimulus

An important part of persistent pain is the ability of the nervous system to modify its function (Rowbotham, Kidd, and Porreca 2006). This phenomenon is called *neuronal plasticity*. This can lead to a phenomenon called peripheral sensitization when nociceptors are sensitized. This sensitization is a result of inflammation when tissue is injured and inflammatory mediators such as bradykinin, histamine, serotonin, adenosine, and nitric oxide are all released from damaged tissue. Cytokines and growth factors are recruited to the site, and an increased inflammatory response is produced. This sensitizes the peripheral neurons, leading to a condition where nonpainful touch and pressure become painful.

There are several other physiologic actions that help either decrease, increase, or prolong pain stimulus. The first is called *wind-up*. This phenomenon is the result of repeated assault on afferent nerves, creating a greatly enhanced response and activity level in the central nervous system. Examples of disease states where wind-up becomes very problematic are osteoarthritis and rheumatoid arthritis (Rowbotham, Kidd, and Porreca 2006). The wind-up allows even normal tissue to become extremely sensitive to pressure in areas that are not identified as painful.

As a consequence of wind-up, a phenomenon called central sensitization can occur. This condition is the result of continued transmission of painful stimuli from the periphery, which continually excites spinal neurons. The continued activation of spinal cord neurons results in the development of secondary support systems that continue to help generate the pain stimuli. NMDA receptors are activated as pain continues to be transmitted, thereby helping to maintain and prolong the central sensitization (Dickenson and Besson 2005; Rowbotham, Kidd, and Porecca 2006).

A full discussion of difficult-to-treat pain syndromes related to altered pain processing will be provided in chapters 8 and 9. The case study that follows illustrates how these alterations in neuronal processing can produce a difficult-to-treat pain syndrome.

The following are important elements of the physiologic response to pain stimulus:

- **Neuronal plasticity:** Ability of the nervous system to change or alter its function

- **Wind-up:** Enhanced response to pain stimulus produced by prolonged pain production

- **Peripheral sensitization:** Result of inflammatory process that creates hypersentivity to touch and pressure

- **Central sensitization:** Excitatory process involving spinal nerves produced by continued pain stimuli can persist even after peripheral stimulation is no longer present

Practice exercises

Case study: Mrs. Peters

Mrs. Peters, who is 65 years old, sees her primary care physician after having a painful rash over one side of her chest for several days. She tells the doctor that the pain is there all the time and is so severe that she cannot sleep at night. After examining Mrs. Peters, the doctor finds a vesicular rash over her chest and back on one side of her body. The diagnosis is herpes zoster (or shingles). Three months later, the rash has healed, but Mrs. Peters is still having significant pain in the affected area. She tells the doctors, "I can't stand to wear clothing over the area where that rash was. It just hurts to even think about touching it, and the worst thing is the burning. It just goes on forever. Will I ever get better?"

Rationale

Mrs. Peters is suffering from postherpetic neuralgia (PHN), a difficult-to-treat neuropathic pain syndrome. The continued pain stimulus caused her body to activate some of the abnormal responses to pain.

1. **What types of pain is Mrs. Peters experiencing, and why is touch so painful for her?**
   Mrs. Peters has both persistent and neuropathic pain. She is also experiencing allodynia and hyperalgesia (see Chapter 1). With the continued input from the injured peripheral neurons and the continued inflammatory effect at the site of the tissue damage, the pain impulses from the periphery continue to activate the spinal neurons. The resulting wind-up and peripheral sensitization have caused even normal touch to be painful. This is a very difficult-to-treat pain syndrome that will require a combination of opioid pain medications and medication to treat neuropathic pain. The medications for this type of condition are discussed in Chapter 4.

2. Search the Web for neuropathic syndromes, such as postherpetic neuralgia, and find what types of treatments are indicated. Search for Complex Regional Pain Syndrome (CRPS), phantom limb pain, post thoracotomy pain, or post mastectomy pain as examples. Determine how the effect of altered pain transmission produces these painful conditions.

Pain assessment

Learning objectives

After reading this chapter, the participant should be able to

- identify the elements of pain assessment

- describe common barriers to pain assessment

Pain is subjective, so measuring pain intensity and other factors influencing pain has always been problematic for nurses. Unlike, say, blood pressure or hemoglobin, pain does not have an objective measure. When measuring blood pressure, there is a numeric equivalent that the patient has no control over. Blood pressure can be 90/60, 120/80, or 180/90, but the values are concrete numbers. Hemoglobin is the same. The blood taken from the patient is sent to a laboratory where a machine measures the amount of hemoglobin in the sample, giving a numeric equivalent.

For pain, however, nurses are taught to ask the patient about the pain, rely on self report for patients who are able to provide one, and act on the patient's report of pain intensity and other descriptors. Many healthcare providers have difficulty believing patients when they report pain, which leads to undertreatment of pain for many patients (Donovan, Dillon, and McGuire 1987; Harrison 1991; Berry et al 2006). This is particularly true for patients with chronic or persistent pain. This chapter provides an overview of pain assessment and a discussion of the barriers to pain assessment.

How to assess pain

Pain assessment is not a "one size fits all" process. Each patient's pain is experienced in many ways and on many levels. Since self report of pain is the accepted method for assessing pain intensity, nurses must rely on the patient to provide a description of the pain and put a value on the intensity of the pain, which can be very confusing. One patient's "discomfort" may be another person's "agonizing" pain. Understanding the importance of adequate pain assessment can help nurses become more proficient in assessing pain in patients.

When pain is not assessed appropriately it can lead to undertreated pain. Undertreated pain can cause numerous problems:

- **Undertreated acute pain** can cause serious medical complications (such as pneumonia and deep vein thrombosis), may impair recovery, and can potentially progress to a difficult-to-treat chronic pain condition (APS 2003, D'Arcy 2007)

- **Undertreated chronic pain** can limit daily activities, increase disability, negatively affect quality of life, create suffering, increase the risk for suicide (Harwood 2006, Tang & Crane 2006), and cause anxiety, depression, anger, and fear (Berry et al 2006).

Pain tip

A significant adverse effect of undertreated acute pain is the possibility of progression to a chronic pain syndrome that is much more difficult to treat (Berry et al 2006). For example, undertreatment of pain from injuries—such as crush injuries—can lead to Complex Regional Pain Syndrome (CRPS) (D'Arcy 2007). Nurses should recognize this risk for patients who continue to report severe pain levels following surgical procedures or injuries.

Pain Management: Evidence-Based Tools and Techniques for Nursing Professionals

Tips when assessing for pain

To avoid some of the sequelae of undertreated pain, it is important for nurses to understand how to assess pain. The elements of a pain assessment include the following:

- **Location:** Have patients point to where the pain is located on their bodies.

- **Intensity:** Using a simple Likert-type scale (0 for no pain and 10 for the worst pain), ask patients to indicate the intensity of the pain.

- **Duration:** Patients should be asked the following questions: "When did the pain start?", "How long does the pain last?", and "Is there anything that you remember that caused the pain to start, such as an injury?" These questions will indicate how long the patient has been in pain and identify any unrelieved or undertreated pain.

- **Description:** Ask patients to describe the pain using verbal descriptors such as burning, shooting, achy, and dull. Do not supply words to patients; allow them to describe the pain in their own words.

- **Aggravating or alleviating factors:** Ask patients what makes the pain better and what makes the pain worse, to elicit information about what they have tried to relieve pain and what modalities might help (e.g., heat or cold).

- **Functional impairment:** Pain is dynamic and increases with activity (Dahl 2006). Ask patients how pain interferes with their activities. Can they walk as far as they used to? Can they take care of themselves at home, or does the pain make it impossible? Is sleep affected? These questions tell you how much the pain is impairing their ability to function.

- **Pain goal:** Set a reasonable pain goal with patients. Ask them what level of pain relief would be acceptable to them, given the pain they are experiencing and the cause of the pain.

(D'Arcy 2003, ASPMN 2002, JCAHO 2001, JCAHO 2000)

There are certain "red flags" that should not be missed when performing a pain assessment. For patients whose main complaint is pain, be sure to also assess the patient for

- significant weight loss or pain that worsens at night and does not resolve at rest while lying down. This may indicate that the source of the pain is a malignancy.

- neurologic symptoms that accompany pain, such as bowel or bladder incontinence, motor weakness in the lower extremities, or any loss of function in extremities, which could signal a spinal cord impairment.

(D'Arcy 2006)

Remember that pain is as important as taking vital signs; the American Pain Society suggests that pain assessment should be considered "the 5th vital sign"(APS 2003, Berry 2006). In addition, the American Society of Perianesthesia Nurses (ASPAN) recommends that pain should be frequently assessed in the postanesthesia care unit (ASPAN 2003).

Consider Peter, who is a patient with chronic pain.

Assessing Peter's pain

Case study: Peter

Peter, age 42, tells you about his pain. "I was just riding my bike down the street one night and all of a sudden the car just hit me. I was rushed to the hospital with two fractured legs and some back damage. I don't remember much of the first days in the hospital. It is all a blur, and I was on a lot of pain medications. Later they had me on a patient controlled analgesia (PCA) pump for over a week while I was having surgeries. During my rehabilitation they changed me over to oral pain medications that really didn't do much for the pain. I couldn't always do my physical therapy because of the pain; it just hurt too badly. Now I still have some residual pain and this nasty, burning, tingling pain in my right foot that just won't go away. The neuropathic pain medication helps some. I always rate the pain at least 8/10. I can't wear shoes, and walking is really hard. It's been over a year. Won't this pain ever get better? I would be happy to see the pain below a 5/10."

- **Location:** right foot

- **Intensity:** 8/10

- **Duration:** > than 1 year

- **Description:** burning, painful, tingling

- **Aggravating factors:** walking, shoes

- **Alleviating factors:** a neuropathic pain medication

- **Functional impairment:** can't walk any distance; wearing shoes is hard

- **Pain goal:** 5/10 or less

Peter's pain is simple to assess if the right questions are asked, which is the case for most patients. By asking the right questions and waiting for the patient to supply the information, a good pain assessment does not need to take a long time. Having someone on the clinic staff or a nursing assistant screen patients for pain by asking for a pain intensity rating can identify patients who are having pain control problems. The person doing the screening should have parameters that indicate when the nurse should be notified of a patient's pain rating for further assessment, such as any patient reporting pain of greater than 5/10.

Pain tip

Remember to document all the elements of the pain assessment. If it is not documented, then it is considered to not have happened (Camp & O'Sullivan 1987).

Barriers to pain assessment

There are several different types of barriers that prevent nurses from performing a good pain assessment. Some are related to the healthcare system, and some are related to bias demonstrated by healthcare providers. The fragmenting of modern healthcare, failure to comply with standards that make pain relief a priority, and time constraints on staff all make pain assessment difficult (Berry et al 2006).

Healthcare providers also bring their own prejudices and bias to practice settings (Harrison 1991). Although the single best indicator of pain intensity is patient report, many healthcare providers still have difficulty accepting the patient's report of pain as valid (Grossman et al 1991, Paice et al 1991, Drayer et al 1999, Donovan et al 1987, Berry et al 2006). It is incumbent on nurses and other healthcare providers to honor patients' reports of pain and accept them as the best estimate that patients can provide. It is unacceptable to ask a patient about pain and then minimize the report or attempt to discredit or lower a patient's report of pain to make it seem less significant (Camp and O'Sullivan 1987).

When pain assessment is not done accurately or completely, the patient will suffer. There are many studies that indicate reluctance to prescribe opioids for pain relief in patients is related to either clinician fears of addicting patients, fears of respiratory depression, or unwillingness to accept patient report as a valid report of pain intensity (Marks and Sachar 1973, Apfelbaum 2003, Donovan et al 1987, Choiniere et al 1990, Harrison A. 1991, Watt-Watson 1987).

Regulatory and accreditation focus on pain

Because of these issues, in 1992 and 1994 the Agency for Health Care Policy and Research (AHCPR) recognized the barriers and issues surrounding pain assessment and tried to call attention to the need for better pain relief for patients by issuing Clinical Practice Guidelines for acute and cancer pain management. Unfortunately, little changed clinically for patients. Since 2000, The Joint Commission has been focusing on pain, pain assessment, and adequate pain relief for patients.

 Pain Management: Evidence-Based Tools and Techniques for Nursing Professionals

Currently, The Joint Commission mandates that organizations comply with the following requirements:

- Patients have a right to have their pain assessed and reassessed regularly

- Patients have a right to adequate pain treatment

- Language cannot be a barrier to pain assessment and treatment

- Patients should be involved in their plan of care, including pain management

- Patients should be educated about their pain medication and any potential side effects

Undertreating pain makes facilities liable

Failure to assess pain can lead to undertreatment of pain, which can have significant legal implications in addition to patient-related consequences. In a much-discussed 1990 case, Estate of Henry James vs. Hillhaven Corporation, a North Carolina jury awarded $15 million to the estate of the plaintiff for compensatory and punitive damages (Angolara 1991, D'Arcy 2003). In this case, a terminal oncology patient with a pathological femur fracture was stabilized on morphine elixir. When the patient was transferred to a second facility, the admission nurse indicated in her assessment that she felt the patient was receiving too much morphine. Consequently, another medication was substituted for some of the subsequent morphine doses. The patient experienced unrelieved pain and died shortly thereafter.

As a direct result of the nursing assessment on admission to the second facility, in a second suit the North Carolina Department of Human Resources fined that facility for patient endangerment and found the nurse liable (Pasero 2001). There have been other cases where undertreated pain has been cited as evidence of elder abuse (LaGanaga 2001, Yi 2001).

Nurses' vital role

Nurses play an important role in pain assessment. Patients trust that nurses will help them with their pain and are willing to give the nurse all the information they need for an adequate assessment. By learning the important aspects of pain assessment and helping patients to report their pain effectively, pain management care for patients can be improved and can direct the choice of options for care.

Practice exercises

1. Using the elements of pain assessment (see "Tips when assessing for pain"), list the pieces of the patient report that fit into each category.

Case study: Susanna Rollins

Susanna, 32, has been coming to the outpatient clinic regularly for the last 18 months and complaining of pain "all over." She has been having difficulty sleeping at night and feels depressed. She tells you that she "just can't get herself straightened out emotionally." She feels too young to have her joints ache and takes Tylenol for the pain, but it really does not help. She has tried heat and cold packs with little relief, and she recently went for an evaluation by the clinic psychologist. The psychologist gave her a prescription for Cyclobenzaprine (Flexeril), which has helped her muscle soreness, and an antidepressant.

Susanna reports that her feet, ankles, and hips hurt, and she rates the pain at 5/10, though it is worse at night when she can't sleep. She is worried about her future, since it is difficult for her to keep working. She would like the pain to be around a 3/10 if she has to live with it. She also says she could stand the pain if she just knew what was wrong with her.

Today Susanna's physician tells her she has fibromyalgia.

Practice exercises (cont.)

Pain assessment:

- **Location:** Feet, hips, knees, all over

- **Pain intensity:** 5/10, worse at night

- **Duration:** 18 months

- **Description:** Aching

- **Aggravating:** Having to go to work, uncertainty of diagnosis

- **Alleviating:** Medication

- **Functional Impairment:** Feels too old for her age and can't work consistently

- **Pain Goal:** 3/10

The American Pain Society has Fibromyalgia Pain Guidelines for managing the pain associated with this syndrome. The highest recommendations are for cyclobenzaprine (Flexeril) or amitriptyline (Elavil). Opioids are not recommended for pain relief, but tramadol (Ultram) has good evidence for use with pain flares. Other options with strong research support include cardiovascular exercise, cognitive behavioral therapy (CBT), patient education, and multidisciplinary therapy, such as combining exercise and CBT. (APS 2005, D'Arcy & McCarberg 2005).

Pain assessment tools and scales

Learning objectives

After reading this chapter, the participant should be able to

- discuss various tools used for pain assessment

- identify pain assessment tools for specialty populations

Assessment is best performed using reliable and valid pain assessment scales and tools. This chapter

provides examples of some of the more commonly used scales and tools for both acute and chronic

pain, as well as those used for pediatric patients and patients with cognitive impairment or in critical

care areas.

Standard pain assessment tools: Unidimensional tools

Some of the earliest pain assessment tools are one-dimensional pain scales, which were designed to

measure pain intensity alone. Examples of this type of scale include the Visual Analog Scale (VAS),

the Verbal Descriptor Scale (VDS), and the standard 0 to 10 Numeric Pain Intensity Scale (NPI).

A systematic review of 164 journal articles on pain indicates that single item ratings of pain intensity

are valid and reliable measures of pain intensity (Jensen 2003).

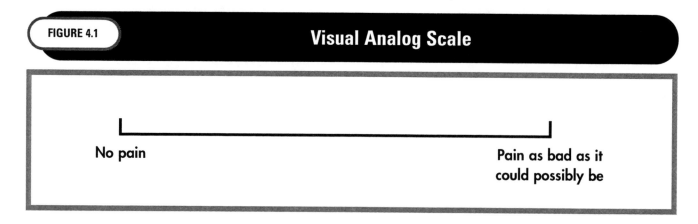

FIGURE 4.1 — Visual Analog Scale

No pain

Pain as bad as it could possibly be

The Visual Analog Scale (VAS) is a 100-millimeter line with "no pain" on one end and "pain as bad as it can be" at the other end. This scale is a very simple form of assessment. Patients are expected to mark on the line the amount of pain they are experiencing.

Patients with visual impairment find this scale difficult to use, and some elderly patients have difficulty marking on the line (Herr 1993, AHCPR 1994, D'Arcy 2003).

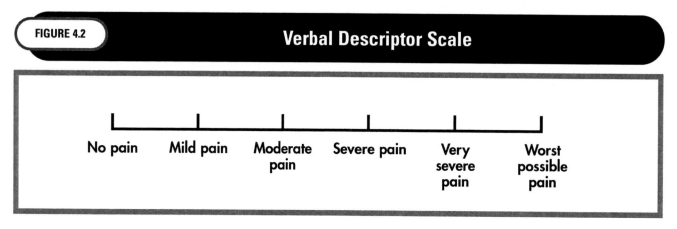

FIGURE 4.2 — Verbal Descriptor Scale

No pain   Mild pain   Moderate pain   Severe pain   Very severe pain   Worst possible pain

The Verbal Descriptor Scale (VDS) uses words such as "no pain," "moderate pain," or "worst possible pain" to help patients describe pain intensity. To use this scale, patients must be able to understand the use of the words and their meanings.

Feldt, Ryden, and Miles (1998) found a 73% completion rate using this scale with a group of cognitively impaired patients. Additionally, some adults prefer using words to describe pain rather than numbers (Herr 1993, D'Arcy 2003).

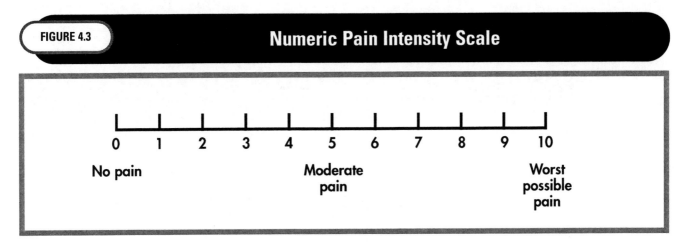

FIGURE 4.3 · Numeric Pain Intensity Scale

The most commonly used one-dimensional pain scale is the Numeric Pain Intensity Scale (NPI), also called the Numeric Rating Scale (NRS). This scale is made up of a horizontal line with the beginning point marked 0, or "no pain," and the opposite end marked 10, or "worst possible pain." Patients are asked to rate their pain from 0 to 10, choosing the number that best represents the intensity of the pain they are experiencing. Generally the pain in the 1–3 range is considered mild pain, 4–6 indicates moderate pain, and 7–10 is the highest level, or severe level, of pain.

This scale is useful for assessing efficacy of pain interventions. For example, by asking the patient for a numeric rating prior to pain medication and then asking the pain rating after half an hour or one hour, healthcare providers can measure the efficacy of the medication. A decrease of three points on the NPI is considered to be significant (Gordon et al, 2004)

There is no right or wrong number for patients to report. The nurse should ask the patient to rate the pain, and he or she should believe the number the patient reports.

Using standard pain assessment scales

For acute pain, standard pain assessment scales work fairly well. But for patients with chronic pain who live with daily pain, numeric scales are more difficult to use. A better way for nurses to gauge improvement is to ask patients with chronic pain what level they experience on a daily basis. For these patients, success with pain management may need to be measured by the increase in a patient's functionality, rather than by the decrease in pain intensity (Pasero & McCaffery 2004).

Visual pain assessment tools and combined pain assessment scales

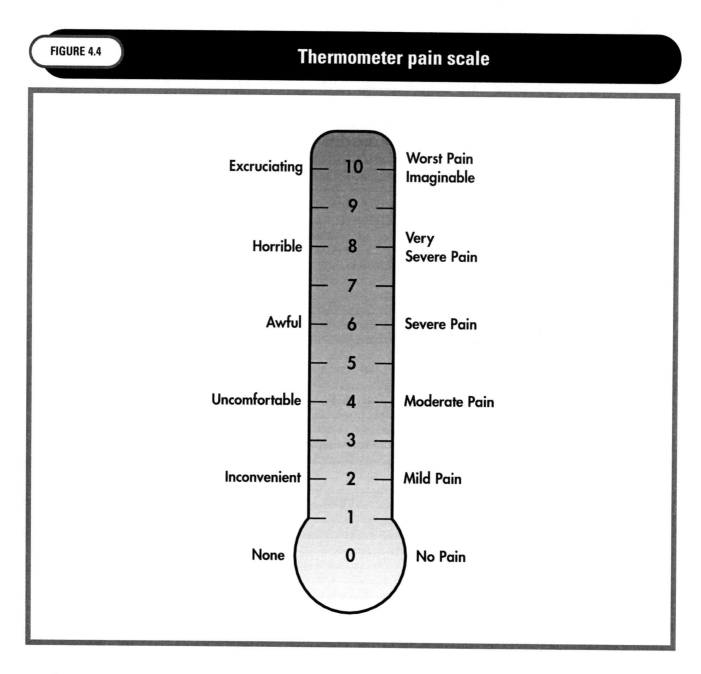

FIGURE 4.4 — **Thermometer pain scale**

Excruciating	10	Worst Pain Imaginable
	9	
Horrible	8	Very Severe Pain
	7	
Awful	6	Severe Pain
	5	
Uncomfortable	4	Moderate Pain
	3	
Inconvenient	2	Mild Pain
	1	
None	0	No Pain

Some patients rate pain more easily when given a picture of the pain scale. The combined scale may use a grayscale (light to dark) or color (blue for less pain and red for more pain) and arranges the numbers in ascending order. For patients who have difficulty with numeric ratings, the verbal descriptors along the thermometer may help patients determine where the pain they are experiencing should be rated (D'Arcy 2003).

FIGURE 4.5 | **Wong-Baker FACES pain rating scale**

0	1	2	3	4	5
No Hurt	Hurts Little Bit	Hurts Little More	Hurts Even More	Hurts Whole Lot	Hurts Worst

From Hochenberry-Eaton, M., Wilson, D., Winkelstein, M.L. (2005). Wong's Essentials of Pediatric Nursing, *Ed. 7. St. Louis: Mosby, Used with permission. Copyright Mosby.*

The FACES scale was originally developed for use with pediatric patients who are unable to use the numeric pain intensity scale. It has faces that go from happy and smiling (no pain) to sad and tearful (severe pain). The patient is asked to point to the face that best describes the pain they are experiencing. Recently the FACES scale has had concurrent validity established, so that the FACES selection by the patient can be converted to a numeric equivalent (Wong & DiVito-Thomas 2006). This scale has also been validated for use with adults and cognitively impaired patient populations (Wong and Nix 2004).

TIP!

Pain tip

Do not try to match the patient's facial expression to the FACES scale representations. The FACES represent how much pain the patient is experiencing, not the actual facial expression of the patient.

Multidimensional pain scales

There are several multidimensional pain scales that are used to assess patients with chronic pain. These scales use not only a numeric rating of the pain intensity, but also have verbal descriptors, pictures for patients to draw the pain they are experiencing, and indicators of mood. The two pain scales that are most commonly used are the Brief Pain Inventory (BPI) and the Short Form McGill Pain Questionnaire (SF-MPQ)

Brief Pain Inventory

The Brief Pain Inventory (BPI) is a simple and easy-to-use pain instrument for patients with chronic pain. It has been determined to be reliable and valid (Daut et al 1983; Williams, Smith, & Fehnel 2006; Raiche et al 2006; Tittle et al 2003; Tan et al 2004), and it has been translated into many languages (Ger et al 1999, Radbruch et al 1999, Mystakidou 2002, Klepstad 2002). Clinically, it is designed to be used either as a self-report format or as an interview.

The BPI has a pain rating scale, a body diagram to locate the pain, a functional assessment, and questions related to pain medication efficacy. It was originally designed to assess pain in cancer patients, but it has been used with a variety of patient populations who are experiencing chronic pain. Since this scale is more complex to use, the patient must be functioning at a high enough level to understand the questions and provide more detailed information.

FIGURE 4.6	**Brief Pain Inventory (short form)**

Study ID# _____ Hospital# _____

Do not write above this line

Date: _____ Time: _____

Name: _____

                 Last   First   Middle Initial

1) Throughout our lives, most of us have had pain from time to time (such as minor headaches, sprains, and toothaches). Have you had pain other than these everyday kinds of pain today?

                         1. Yes   2. No

2) On the diagram, shade in the areas where you feel pain. Put an X on the area that hurts the most.

                Right   Left   Left   Right

3) Please rate your pain by circling the one number that best describes your pain at its WORST in the past 24 hours.

0	1	2	3	4	5	6	7	8	9	10
No pain										Pain as bad as you can imagine

4) Please rate your pain by circling the one number that best describes your pain at its LEAST in the past 24 hours.

0	1	2	3	4	5	6	7	8	9	10
No pain										Pain as bad as you can imagine

FIGURE 4.6 **Brief Pain Inventory (short form)** (cont.)

5) Please rate your pain by circling the one number that best describes your pain on the AVERAGE.

0	1	2	3	4	5	6	7	8	9	10

No pain   Pain as bad as you can imagine

6) Please rate your pain by circling the one number that tells how much pain you have RIGHT NOW.

0	1	2	3	4	5	6	7	8	9	10

No pain   Pain as bad as you can imagine

7) What treatments or medications are you receiving for your pain?

8) In the past 24 hours, how much relief have pain treatments or medications provided? Please circle the one percentage that most shows how much RELIEF you have received.

0%	10%	20%	30%	40%	50%	60%	70%	80%	90%	100%

No relief   Complete relief

9) Circle the one number that describes how, during the past 24 hours, pain has interfered with your:
   A. General activity:

0	1	2	3	4	5	6	7	8	9	10

Does not interfere   Completely interferes

   B. Mood:

0	1	2	3	4	5	6	7	8	9	10

Does not interfere   Completely interferes

   C. Walking ability:

0	1	2	3	4	5	6	7	8	9	10

Does not interfere   Completely interferes

FIGURE 4.6   **Brief Pain Inventory (short form)** (cont.)

D. Normal work (includes both work outside the home and housework):

0	1	2	3	4	5	6	7	8	9	10

Does not
interfere

Completely
interferes

E. Relations with other people:

0	1	2	3	4	5	6	7	8	9	10

Does not
interfere

Completely
interferes

F. Sleep:

0	1	2	3	4	5	6	7	8	9	10

Does not
interfere

Completely
interferes

G. Enjoyment of life:

0	1	2	3	4	5	6	7	8	9	10

Does not
interfere

Completely
interferes

Reprinted by permission: Copyright 1991, Charles S. Cleeland, Ph.D. Pain Research Group.

FIGURE 4.7

Short-Form McGill Pain Questionnaire

Patient's name: _____   Date: _____

	None	Mild	Moderate	Severe
Throbbing	0) _____	1) _____	2) _____	3) _____
Shooting	0) _____	1) _____	2) _____	3) _____
Stabbing	0) _____	1) _____	2) _____	3) _____
Sharp	0) _____	1) _____	2) _____	3) _____
Cramping	0) _____	1) _____	2) _____	3) _____
Gnawing	0) _____	1) _____	2) _____	3) _____
Hot/burning	0) _____	1) _____	2) _____	3) _____
Aching	0) _____	1) _____	2) _____	3) _____
Heavy	0) _____	1) _____	2) _____	3) _____
Tender	0) _____	1) _____	2) _____	3) _____
Splitting	0) _____	1) _____	2) _____	3) _____
Tiring/exhausting	0) _____	1) _____	2) _____	3) _____
Sickening	0) _____	1) _____	2) _____	3) _____
Fearful	0) _____	1) _____	2) _____	3) _____
Punishing/cruel	0) _____	1) _____	2) _____	3) _____

VAS |_____|

No pain   Worst possible pain

PPI

0	No pain	_____
1	Mild	_____
2	Discomforting	_____
3	Distressing	_____
4	Horrible	_____
5	Excruciating	_____

The Short-Form McGill Pain Questionnaire (SF-MPQ). Descriptors 1-11 represent the sensory dimension of pain experience and 12-15 represent the affective dimension. Each descriptor is ranked on an intensity scale of 0 = none, 1 = mild, 2 = moderate, 3 = severe. The Present Pain Intensity (PPI) of the standard Long-Form McGill Pain Questionnaire (LF-MPQ) and the visual analog scale (VAS) are also included to provide overall intensity scores.

McGill Pain Questionnaire

The McGill Pain Questionnaire (MPQ) has both a long form and a short form, but the short form is used more often, because it covers the most important information and is easier to use. The original version of the pain instrument had three classes of verbal descriptors that were weighted and scored, a body diagram to locate the pain, and a pain intensity scale. In the short form, the pain descriptors are listed and divided by dimensions of the pain experience, and there is a visual analog scale to rate the intensity of the pain (Melzack 1975, 1987; McDonald & Weiskopf 2001; Chok 1998; McIntyre et al 1995; Graham 1980; Wilkie 1990).

Both the long and short form of the MPQ have been used both clinically and for research. The MPQ has been translated into several different languages and has been found to be both valid and reliable (Mystakidou 2002). It has been used in many different scenarios, such as measuring post-procedural pain and experimentally induced pain, and in a large number of medical and surgical areas with children over the age of 12. The one drawback to this pain instrument is its inability to translate the meaning of the verbal descriptors chosen by the patients into words that are more descriptive of syndromes (Gracely 1992, Graham et al 1980).

Pain assessment in specialty populations

Pain scale for infants: CRIES

The CRIES scale is one of several pain rating scales that can be used with infants who obviously cannot self-report pain. This scale uses physiologic indicators to assess behaviors indicative of pain. The key elements are the following:

- Crying

- Requires oxygen

- Increased vital signs

- Expression

- Sleeplessness

This scale rates and scores behavior, with a higher score indicative of more distress and pain. The CRIES scale is designed specifically for neonates, but there are other pain scales that can be used for pediatrics. One is the FLACC scale, which uses the elements of faces, legs, activity, cry, and consolability (D'Arcy 2003).

| FIGURE 4.8 | **CRIES neonatal postop-pain measurement score** |

	0	1	2
Crying	No	High pitched	Inconsolable
Requires O2 for Sat >95	No	<30%	>30%
Increased vital signs	HR and BP = or < preop	HR or BP increased <20% of preop	HR or BP increased >20% of preop
Expression	None	Grimace	Grimace/Grunt
Sleepless	No	Wakes at frequent intervals	Constantly awake

Neonatal pain assessment tool developed at the University of Missouri-Columbia, Copyright S. Krechel, MD, and J. Bildner, RNC, CNS. Used with permission.

 Pain Management: Evidence-Based Tools and Techniques for Nursing Professionals

FIGURE 4.8 **CRIES neonatal postop-pain measurement score** (cont.)

Coding tips for using CRIES

Crying

The characteristic cry of pain is *high pitched*.
If no cry or cry which is not high pitched **score 0**
If cry high pitched but baby is easily consoled **score 1**
If cry is high pitched and baby is inconsolable **score 2**

Requires O2 for sat > 95%

Look for *changes* in oxygenation. Babies experiencing pain manifest decreases in oxygenation as measured by TCo2 or oxygen saturation.

If no oxygen is required **score 0**
If < 30% O2 is required **score 1**
If > 30% is required **score 2**

(Consider other causes of changes in oxygenation: atelectasis, pneumothorax, over sedation, etc.)

Increased vital signs

*Note: Take blood pressure last as this may wake child, causing difficulty with other assessments.
Use baseline preop parameters from a nonstressed period.
Multiply baseline HR x 0.2 then add this to baseline HR to determine the HR, which is 20% over baseline.
Do likewise for BP. Use mean BP.
If HR and BP are both unchanged or less than baseline, **score 0**
If HR or BP is increased, but increase is <20% of baseline, **score 1**
If either one is increased >20% over baseline, **score 2**

Expression

The facial expression most often associated with pain is a grimace. This may be characterized by brow lowering, eyes squeezed shut, deepening of the nasolabial furrow, open lips and mouth.
If no grimace is present, **score 0**
If grimace alone is present, **score 1**
If grimace and noncry vocalization grunt are present, **score 2**

Sleepless

This parameter is scored based upon the infant's state during the hour preceding this recorded score.
If the child has been continuously asleep, **score 0**
If he/she has awakened at frequent intervals, **score 1**
If he/she has been awake constantly, **score 2**

Pain tip

Pain scales are meant to assess pain in the patient populations they were designed for. Adult pain scales should not be used for pediatric patients and, conversely, pediatric pain scales should not be used for adults unless validity and reliability have been established. To do so alters the pain assessment and, consequently, the patient's pain cannot be reliably assessed.

Using behavioral pain scales

Using behavioral pain scales is controversial. It is widely accepted that the standard for pain assessment is the patient's self report of pain. However, some patient populations are unable to self-report pain. Although it is very early in the development of behavioral pain scales, there is no single scale that will work for these populations. Assigning a numeric equivalent to the behaviors so it can be converted to a numeric pain intensity (NPI) rating is sometimes not possible (Herr et al 2006). The lack of a number means that it is identified as present, but there is no way to quantify the pain and nurses have no trigger to treat it. When considering the use of a behavioral pain scale, choose one that fits the patient you are trying to assess.

When assessing pain in patients who cannot report their pain, the important elements are the following:

• Attempt a self report

• Search for potential causes of pain

• Observe patient behaviors

• Surrogate reporting by family or caregivers of pain and behavior/activity changes

• Attempt an analgesic trial

(Herr et al 2006)

Checklist of Non-verbal Pain Indicators

The Checklist of Non-verbal Pain Indicators (CNPI) is a list of six behaviors that have been determined to demonstrate pain (Feldt 2000; Feldt, Ryden, & Miles 1998). These six behaviors are

- vocalizations

- facial grimacing

- bracing

- rubbing

- restlessness

- vocal complaints

These behaviors were determined in a study that compared a sample of patients who were cognitively impaired to patients who were not cognitively impaired (Feldt 2000).

This checklist tool was designed for use with older, cognitively impaired adults in acute care settings (Herr 2006).

Additional behaviors that are indicative of pain are listed in the American Geriatrics Society's guideline for persistent pain in older persons (2002):

- **Verbalizations:** Moaning, calling out, asking for help, groaning

- **Facial expressions:** Grimacing, frowning, wrinkled forehead, distorted expressions

- **Body movements:** Rigid tense body posture, guarding, rocking, fidgeting, pacing, massaging the painful area

- **Changes in interpersonal interactions:** Aggression, combative behavior, resisting care, disruptive, withdrawn

- **Changes in activity patterns or routines:** Refusing food, appetite changes, increase in rest or sleep, increased wandering

- **Mental status changes:** Crying, tears, increased confusion, irritability or distress

Although behaviors are not the ideal method for assessing pain in nonverbal patients, these behaviors have been identified as indicators that pain is present. Using these behaviors or changes in behaviors can help to identify pain in patients who cannot self-report pain.

Pain Assessment in Advanced Dementia

The Pain Assessment in Advanced Dementia (PAINAD) assessment tool was designed to assess pain in patients with dementia or Alzheimer's disease who cannot self-report pain (Lane 2003). The scale consists of five items:

- Breathing

- Negative vocalizations

- Facial expression

- Body language

- Consolability

One of the conceptual problems with the PAINAD scale is that it relies on caregivers' assessment of pain intensity, which is not currently seen as accurate (Herr 2006). This tool uses some of the recommendations from the American Geriatrics Society, but not all of them, and thus it is seen as

FIGURE 4.9

Pain Assessment IN Advanced Dementia (PAINAD)

Pain Assessment IN Advanced Dementia
PAINAD

	0	1	2	Score
Breathing Independent of vocalization	Normal	Occasional labored breathing. Short period of hyperventilation	Noisy labored breathing. Long period of hyperventilation. Cheyne-stokes respirations	
Negative Vocalization	None	Occasional moan or groan. Low level speech with a negative or disapproving quality	Repeated troubled calling out. Loud moaning or groaning. Crying	
Facial expression	Smiling, or inexpressive	Sad. Frightened. Frown	Facial grimacing	
Body Language	Relaxed	Tense. Distressed pacing. Fidgeting	Rigid. Fists clenched. Knees pulled up. Pulling or pushing away. Striking out	
Consolability	No need to console	Distracted or reassured by voice or touch	Unable to console, distract or reassure	
				TOTAL

Developed at the New England Geriatric Research Education and Clinical Center, EN Rogers Memorial Veterans Hospital, Bedford, MA. Reference: Warden, V., Hurley, A.C., & Volicer, L. (2003). "Development and psychometric evaluation of the Pain Assessment in Advanced Dementia (PAINAD) Scale." *Journal of the American Medical Directors Association* 4: 9-15. Used with permission.

less comprehensive than perhaps is necessary for assessing pain in more complex cases involving demented older patients (Herr 2006).

However, as a quick and easy-to-use clinical assessment tool, it provides a base assessment, and the tool should be developed and studied further. Nurses need to be aware of the tool, since it will likely become more popular as it is developed further.

Payen Behavioral Pain Scale for intubated patients

One very difficult group of patients to assess for pain is the intensive care unit (ICU) patient who is sedated and intubated. The Thunder Project II study was a large national study conducted by the American Association of Critical Care Nurses, where thousands of patients were asked about pain during procedures such as suctioning and turning. The results from the study have been used as a benchmark for pain in critical care. Data from this study tells us that some of the most routine nursing practices can result in pain for patients. For example, simply turning a patient in a bed received a ranking of 4 to 5 out of 10 on a numeric pain scale (Puntillo et al 2001).

Payen developed a pain assessment tool specifically for intubated ICU patients. It contains a three-point assessment and elements that fit the patient population (2001):

1. Facial expressions

2. Upper limb movement

3. Compliance with ventilation

The Payen assessment tool can help you derive a pain rating for intubated patients by examining the three behaviors that correspond to an identified pain stimulus when the patient is sedated with medications such as propofol (Diprovan).

The Payen study used three different groups of ICU patients who were either mildly, moderately, or heavily sedated and intubated, respectively. Findings indicated that the three behaviors correlated with a numeric pain intensity scale (Payen 2001, Purdum & D'Arcy 2006).

This scale allows pain to be assessed in patients who previously were thought to be unassessable. An observation tool developed by Gelinas et al (2006) had similar findings related to the ability to determine pain behaviors in sedated, intubated ICU patients. The tool allows for pain intensity to be estimated, which can provide a trigger for treatment. However, like all behavioral pain scales, this scale also needs more study and development to ensure that the elements being used for assessment truly represent pain intensity in this population.

Final word on pain assessment

- Remember that all patients have the right to have their pain assessed. This means infants, children, ICU patients, and older patients with dementia all need to have an assessment for pain.

- The pain assessment is more than a number. It is a holistic assessment that covers elements that are difficult to tease out, such as the meaning of the pain to the patient.

- Believe what patients tell you about their pain.

- Use a pain scale that fits the patient you are assessing.

Practice exercises

1. Log on to the Web site of the American Geriatrics Society (*www.americangeriatrics.org*) and read the Guideline for Treatment of Persistent Pain in Older Adults. Visit the Web site of the American Society for Pain Management Nursing (ASPMN) (*www.aspmn.org*) and read the position statement on Pain Assessment in Non-verbal Patients.

   Was the information useful? Did you learn something new about assessing pain in older adults? Were you aware of the behavioral pain scales that are being used? Did you find a behavioral pain scale that you think you can use in your practice?

2. Look at the patient in this case study and see if you can assess the patient's pain.

Case Study: John Jones

John is a patient with Alzheimer's disease. He is usually very pleasant and he smiles a lot. He takes his meals with the other patients and can feed himself. Today he is very angry and pushes you away when you try to get him up in the morning. He does not want to eat and becomes very irritable when you continue to try to get him up. He moans to himself and rubs his leg. When you look at his leg you see a large reddened area with swelling. You don't know what happened, and he can't tell you about his pain.

A. **What were the indicators of pain?**
Irritable, change in behavior from happy to grumpy, won't eat or get out of bed, moaning and rubbing leg.

B. **Can you rate the intensity of the pain?**
No, but there is a significant change in the patient's behavior, and he is moaning.

C. **What pain scale would be suitable for assessing this patient's pain?**
PAINAD.

D. **Would a trial of pain medication be indicated for this patient?**
Yes.

Pain medications

Learning objectives

After reading this chapter, the participant should be able to

- review The Joint Commission's recommendations for choosing analgesia

- identify how to select a pain medication using the WHO Analgesic Ladder

- differentiate between medication types: opioids, non-opioids, and adjuvant medications for pain relief

Treating pain

Medications are the most common treatment for pain. However, current reports indicate that pain is still being undertreated (Marks and Sachar et al). In Chapter 3, healthcare providers' bias and unwillingness to believe patients' statements of pain were identified as barriers to adequate pain relief (Dillon, Donovan, McGuire 1987; Harrison 1991; Berry et al 2006). Lack of knowledge about prescribing and combining medications to treat pain also contribute to undertreated pain (Marks & Sachar). Patient and prescriber fears of addiction limit the use of opioid medication (APS, AAPM, 1997). Additionally, lack of understanding of how to use equianalgesic conversion for medications can lead to undertreatment of pain (Anderson et al 2001, Ginsberg et al 2003).

Pain tip

Equianalgesic is a term that means equal pain relief. It is used when one medication is converted to another medication or one form of a medication is converted to another route (Anderson et al 2001). For example, 30 milligrams of oral morphine is the equianalgesic equivalent of 10 milligrams of intravenous morphine (APS 2003, ASPMN 2002). Remember that these numeric conversions are based on a one-time, single-dose comparison (APS 2003) and the dose recommendations are useful as a guide only (Anderson et al 2001).

Nurses are in a unique position. They can act as advocates, helping to ensure that patients get a pain medication designed to treat the type of pain they are experiencing. They can use their knowledge to educate other staff about equianalgesic conversion and how to choose the correct pain medication for the pain the patient is reporting. Nurses are not only key to an adequate pain assessment, they are also key to helping patients get a pain medication that works to treat the pain they are experiencing.

How to choose a pain medication

The Joint Commission recommendations

Nurses usually have a choice of several medications, several different routes, and several different doses. The Joint Commission has limited the use of range orders—those orders specifying an open dose and open time frames—and has asked that orders be written with specific doses and time frames. An example of an order that is no longer recommended is, "Percocet one to two tablets every 4 to 6 hours as needed for pain."

A correct order would be "Percocet one tablet every 4 hours as needed for pain."

The Joint Commission has also instituted a requirement that pain be assessed when medication is given and at regular intervals after the medication is administered. Recommended time frames for reassessment are after one hour for oral pain medications and after 30 minutes for intravenous pain medications. Both recommendations are based on the length of time it takes for a medication to be absorbed into a patient's body and provide pain relief (D'Arcy 2006, D'Arcy 2005). The reassessment requirement is one attempt by The Joint Commission to help decrease the undertreatment of pain.

World Health Organization analgesic ladder

Pain medications are not all equal in strength, and each patient can have a different response to a particular medication or dose. Pain medication is a highly individualized type of patient care, and opioids, for example, are not suitable for every patient. To determine what pain medication works best for the patient, you can use a tool such as the World Health Organization (WHO) analgesic ladder to give you a starting point.

Using the analgesic ladder can provide direction for all practitioners about where a medication falls in the analgesic spectrum (Dalton & Youngblood 2000).

Although the WHO ladder was originally developed for use with cancer patients, it is now widely applied for all types of pain. The concept of the ladder is to group the pain medications according to type of pain: mild, moderate, or severe. Although numbers are only a guide to pain intensity, using a grouping of medications for each level provides opportunity for individualizing the medication selection. As always, medication efficacy is an individualized response based on the patient's report of decreased pain.

Pain tip

Mild pain is generally considered to be pain of 1–3 intensity, moderate is 4–7 intensity, and severe pain is 7–10 intensity (APS 2003, ASPMN 2002).

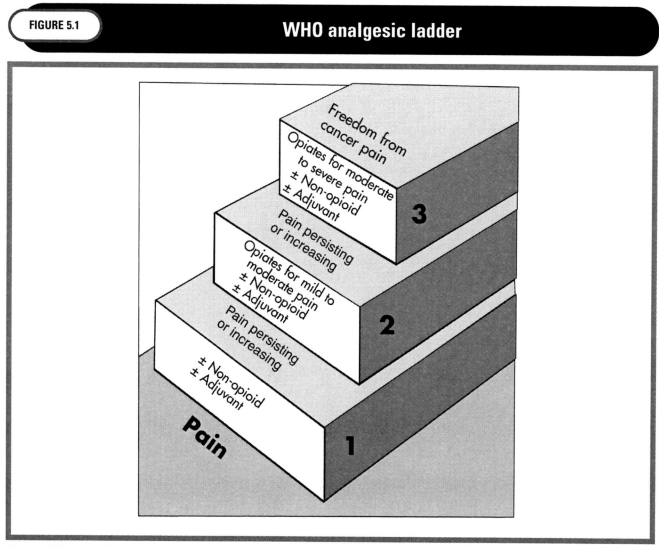

FIGURE 5.1 — **WHO analgesic ladder**

Freedom from cancer pain

Opiates for moderate to severe pain
± Non-opioid
± Adjuvant

3

Pain persisting or increasing

Opiates for mild to moderate pain
± Non-opioid
± Adjuvant

2

Pain persisting or increasing

± Non-opioid
± Adjuvant

Pain

1

Source: WHO, used with permission

When a nurse assesses pain and the patient reports a certain level of pain, looking at the medications available and seeing where they fit on the WHO analgesic ladder can be helpful. For example, if a patient says his or her pain is a 6/10, you would need to have a medication from the moderate pain level or second step of the analgesic ladder. If all you have to offer the patient is Tylenol, you will need to ask the physician for a higher level medication such as Vicodin to help the patient get adequate pain relief.

Level 1 pain medications:
Mild to moderate pain and adjuvant medications

Acetaminophen (Tylenol)

Acetaminophen (Tylenol) is a commonly used pain medication, sold over the counter, that comes in many different forms, tablets, gel caps, and elixirs. The daily maximum dose of Tylenol is 4,000 milligrams; excesses can cause hepatotoxicity. Patients who drink alcohol daily or patients with impaired liver functions should limit their Tylenol use.

Non-Steroidal Anti-Inflammatory Drugs (NSAID)

Non-Selective (NS) Non-Steroidal Anti-Inflammatory Drugs (NSAID) are commonly used medications for pain that are available either as over the counter medications or as prescription strength. They are called non-selective because they affect all types of prostaglandins: those that protect the stomach and those that are found in cardiac and kidney tissue. They are commonly prescribed for inflammatory pain conditions such as arthritis and common musculoskeletal injuries. One of the most common adverse events associated with NSAID use is gastrointestinal (GI) bleeding. Gastric ulcers develop in 30% of all patients on NS NSAIDs within one week, however, no dosage for gastric ulcers and what level of medication may produce an ulcer has been determined (Staats & Wallace 2005). NSAID-related GI bleeds cause 2,600 deaths per year and are responsible for 20,000 hospitalizations annually (Staats and Wallace 2005). Using a proton pump inhibitor such as omeprozole (Prilosec) protects only the upper GI system, leaving the lower GI system vulnerable to ulceration. Chronic alcohol use also increases the risk of GI bleeding and should be discouraged.

> **Notes on pain**
>
> Examples of NS NSAIDs include ibuprofen (Motrin, Advil) and naproxen (Naprosen, Aleve). A complete list of NS NSAID medications is available at the FDA Web site and also includes a patient education guide: *http://www.fda.gov/cder/drug/infopage/COX2/NSAIDmedguide.htm.*

Patients taking NSAIDs who report the following conditions should be instructed to see a physician immediately:

- Black, tarry stools or red blood in the stools

- High blood pressure

- Edema and fluid retention, possibly signaling congestive heart failure

- Vomiting blood

Extremely serious conditions that need emergency intervention include the following:

- Shortness of breath or trouble breathing

- Chest pain

- Weakness in one part or sides of the body

- Slurred speech

- Swelling of the face or throat, signaling anaphylaxis

(FDA 2005, D'Arcy 2005)

COX2 medications

One of the biggest advantages of COX2 medications was the lack of effect on the prostaglandins that protect the stomach lining. This selective effect on the prostaglandins of the stomach did not protect the prostaglandins found in other areas of the body, such as the kidney and heart. Some of the COX2 medications, such as rofecoxib (Vioxx), had a significant effect on the renal prostaglandins, and consequently some patients developed hypertension and had an increased incidence of cardiovascular events. Vioxx (rofecoxib) and Bextra (valdecoxib) are no longer available. Vioxx was withdrawn from the market because of the increased cardiovascular risk, and Bextra was voluntarily removed from the market because of the potential for Stevens Johnson syndrome, a reaction to medications that causes skin to deteriorate and slough.

Celecoxib (Celebrex) is the lone remaining COX2 medication on the market. It is useful for some patients who are good candidates, such as those with inflammatory pain without cardiac conditions. As with all NSAIDs, this medication should be used at the lowest doses and for the shortest time possible.

Recent findings by the Federal Drug Administration (FDA) have found that both types of medications, COX2 and NSAIDs, pose an increased risk for cardiovascular events such as heart attack and stroke, and can decrease the efficacy of aspirin used for cardiac prophylaxis. NS NSAIDs can affect anticoagulants such as coumadin and aspirin since the medications decrease platelet aggregation.

Adjuvant medications

Adjuvant medications have an additive effect for pain relief, but do not by themselves relieve pain. They should be combined with medication at all levels.

Antidepressants

Antidepressants are thought to help pain by acting in the synaptic junction of the nervous system and inhibiting presynaptic uptake of norepinephrine and serotonin (ASPMN 2002). (See Chapter 2 for more on the transmission of pain.) There are several different types of antidepressants used for pain:

- **Tricyclic antidepressants (TCA):** Examples include amitriptyline (Elavil), nortriptyline (Pamelor), and despiramine (Norpramin)

These medications are the oldest antidepressants used for adjunct pain relief: migraine headache, fibromyalgia, and neuropathic pain. Patients taking this type of medication may experience hypotension in the morning, presenting a safety risk for falls. They are not recommended for use by the elderly (APS 2003, Berry 2006).

- **Selective Serotonin Reuptake Inhibitors (SSRI):** Examples include fluoxetine (Prozac), paroxetine (Paxil), sertraline (Zoloft), and citalopram (Celexa)

These are less effective for pain relief than the TCAs, but can be effective for some patients, especially if they have underlying depression. Weight gain is a significant side effect.

- **Selective Serotonin Norepinephrine Reuptake Inhibitors (SNRI):** Examples include duloxetine (Cymbalta), venlafaxine (Effexor), and bupropion (Wellbutrin)

Duloxetine is effective for pain relief in diabetic neuropathy. Wellbutrin is effective for patients with neuropathic pain. As a group, it is more effective for pain relief than SSRIs.

- **Antiseizure medications:** Examples include gabapentin (Neurontin), pregabalin (Lyrica), carbamazepine (Tegretol), oxycarbamazepine (Trileptal), and phenytoin (Dilantin)

These medications are used for neuropathic pain. Tegretol has an indication for trigeminal neuralgia. Trileptal is also used for a variety of painful conditions and has fewer side effects than Tegretol. Neurontin needs to be titrated up to 1,800 milligrams per day to see pain relief. Lyrica is a prodrug of gabapentin (a prodrug is a drug form that precedes the second formulation chemically), so it starts to provide pain relief much sooner than others in this group (APS 2003, Staats et al 2004, Berry et al 2006).

- **Topical medications:** Examples include capsaicin (Zostrix), lidocaine 5% patch (Lidoderm), and analgesic balms (Icy Hot, Ben Gay)

Topical medications are well-tolerated by patients. Zostrix is made from hot peppers and needs a four times per day application schedule for at least four weeks to see the effects (APS 2003). The cream can be irritating to skin and should be applied while the patient is wearing gloves to protect the hands. The Lidoderm patch is designed for use with postherpetic neuralgia (PHN) pain. Up to three patches per day can be applied directly over the painful site on intact skin, for 12 hours on and 12 hours off (Berry et al 2006). Analgesic balms are sold over the counter and provide localized pain relief (APS 2003). Patients should be cautioned not to use a heating pad over the area of application if they are using a mentholated product, to avoid burning the skin.

Level 2 pain medications:
Moderate to severe pain—opioids and adjuvants

Opioids are medications that bind to mu agonist sites throughout the body. Once the medication is released from the systemic uptake, it binds to a specific receptor—mu—that then produces analgesia. There are multiple variations on these mu binding sites, accounting for the variation in patient response to the medication.

Most of the medications in this level are combination medications that use an opioid and acetaminophen. The inclusion of acetaminophen limits how high the doses can be escalated, since the patient's total daily dose cannot exceed 4,000 milligrams of acetaminophen.

Some of the medications at this level are extended-release formulations. These medications do not contain acetaminophen and have actions of 12 to 24 hours. If patients are taking six or more short-acting medications, such as Vicodin or Percocet, then a long-acting medication—such as extended release Vicodin, Avinza, or Oxycontin—should be considered instead. Using an extended-release medication provides a consistent level of pain control (Caldwell et al 2002). Additional short-acting medications such as Vicodin or Percocet can then be provided for breakthrough pain when the patient is more active or has a need for additional pain relief.

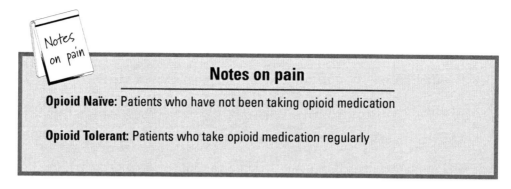

Notes on pain

Opioid Naïve: Patients who have not been taking opioid medication

Opioid Tolerant: Patients who take opioid medication regularly

Codeine containing medications: Tylenol #3. Side effects include constipation; GI upset is common. Used for mild pain relief.

Hydrocodone-containing medications: Vicodin/Lortab, Lortab elixir, extended release Vicodin. Have both short-acting and extended-release forms. The elixir is well tolerated and useful for patients who either have difficulty swallowing tablets or are using feeding tubes.

Oxycodone-containing medications: Percocet, Percodan, Oxycontin, Oxyfast. Oxycontin is the extended-release form of the medication. Oxyfast elixir is well tolerated. These medications provide high-grade pain relief and are commonly used for acute pain management after surgery.

Oxymorphone-containing medications: Opana and OpanaER. These medications have a more extended pain relief action than the above (Adams et al 2004, Adams & Abdieh 2005). When Opana ER, the extended-release form, is used, very little breakthrough medication is needed. Also available in an intravenous form as Neumorphan.

Tramadol: Ultram and Ultram ER. This medication is a combination mu agonist, opioid-like medication combined with an SSRI. This medication is recommended for use in fibromyalgia, and the extended release form is suggested for arthritis pain.

Level 3 pain medications: Severe pain—opioids

Medications in this group are used for severe pain. There is no ceiling on these medications, because they are not combined with acetaminophen. Dosages may be escalated to the level where the patient has pain relief.

Constipation is common with opioid use, and all patients who are using opioids should be given stool softeners and laxatives to use daily. Confusion and hallucination can also occur more commonly in the acute care setting, possibly due to medication combinations or being away from home. Opioids can also cause delirium.

Morphine

Types of morphine include Morphine IR, MS Contin, Kadian, Avinza, and Roxanol. Morphine comes in both an immediate-release form and extended-release forms: MS Contin, Kadian, and Avinza. The biggest adverse effects with morphine are nausea, vomiting, and constipation. The medication can be given IV for acute pain. The elixir is more palatable if a flavoring is added.

Hyromorphone

Hyromorphone (Dilaudid): Dilaudid is a synthetic form of morphine. 0.2 milligrams of Dilaudid is equal to 1 milligram of morphine. This means that pain relief is possible at very small doses, which can help minimize side effects. Dilaudid is available in an oral and IV form.

Fentanyl

Types of Fentanyl include Duragesic patches, Fentora, Fentayl Oralets, and Rapinyl. Fentanyl is a medication than has no oral absorption potential. It degrades in the gastric secretions. It is formulated as a patch, Duragesic, which uses transdermal medication delivery. The medication builds a depot in the subcutaneous fat and lasts for 72 hours. It takes 12 to 18 hours to begin pain relief and as long as 48 hours to build a steady-state medication concentration in the bloodstream. Duragesic patches should never be used for acute pain, because of the time element for action and depletion. Care should be taken to instruct patients who use Duragesic patches to dispose of the used patches in a closed container to avoid accidental overdose by a small child or pet, and no heat should be applied over the patch site because this would cause the medication to be absorbed too rapidly (ISMP 2006). Fentora, an effervescent tablet, Fentanyl oralets, and Rapinyl all rely on buccal absorption of the medication and are designed for use in opioid-tolerant oncology patients for breakthrough pain.

Dolophine

Dolophine (Methadone). This is a medication that provides extended pain relief, with an extended half-life of 22 to 48 hours. Because of the long-action dose, escalations must be done carefully and no more frequently than every three days. The medication comes in a tablet form and an elixir. Caution should be used when increasing doses of methadone. Recent findings indicate there is a potential for cardiac changes that could result in a Torsades syndrome.

Other medications

Mixed agonist-antagonist medications: Examples include Talwin, Nubain, and Buprenex. The mixed agonist-antagonist medications are second-line pain medications. They are used for only mild to moderate pain. They are particularly problematic because they can reverse opioid medications.

Adding extended release medications

Around the clock dosing of pain medication is recommended when pain is present most of the day (Paice 2005, APS 2006). Patients who take short-acting pain medications such as Percocet or Vicodin experience variations in the blood levels of drug and have inconsistent pain relief. In a study of medical patients pain relief was improved with scheduled dosing of pain medications and there was not an increased risk of adverse events (Paice 2005).

When a patient has been taking a pain medication regularly and pain is present most of the day, using an extended-release medication is indicated. Patients with diabetic neuropathy and osteoarthritis had improved pain relief with extended-release formulations (Gimbel 2003, Caldwell 2002).

Problem pain medications

There are two problem pain medications that merit discussion. The first is propoxyphene (Darvocet). Darvocet is a medication designed to treat mild pain. It has 650 milligrams of acetaminophen in each tablet, making it very easy to exceed the daily maximum dose of acetaminophen with just a few tablets per day. In addition, Darvocet has a toxic metabolite called norpropoxyphene that can cause cardiac arrhythmias.

The second problem pain medication is meperidine (Demerol), which is no longer considered a first-line pain medication (APS 2003). Some of the reasons that Demerol has fallen out of favor include the need for high doses to achieve analgesic effect, a high incidence of nausea and sedation, and a neurotoxic metabolite, normeperidine. Normeperidine can build up in the central nervous system and cause seizures (Marinella 1997, APS 2003). It should never be used in patients with impaired renal function or for long-term use, such as with cancer patients. The Joint Commission discourages its use.

Side effects of opioids

Constipation is a common side effect of opioid therapy. This is the only side effect where patients cannot become tolerant. Patients should be instructed to add fiber to their diets, drink fluids, and to use laxatives (such as Senokot) and stool softeners (such as Colace).

Sedation and respiratory depression occur most often at the beginning of opioid therapy. Patients should be observed frequently at the beginning of opioid therapy for signs of sedation. All additional medications that may cause sedation should be eliminated if they are not essential, particularly with older patients.

Pruritis or itching is a common side effect of opioid therapy. This is not an indication of allergy. The itching is caused by histamine release, which responds well to Benadryl or atarax (Vistaril).

Nausea and vomiting can be caused by pain or pain medications. Using an antiemetic regularly can help reduce nausea and vomiting. Reglan can help increase gastric motility, and ondansetron (zofran) and prochloperazine-type antiemetics can help when the cause of nausea is a central chemoreceptor triggered effect.

Pain tip

How to select a pain medication

- Review the case presentation

- Note the type of pain, pain intensity, and any comorbidities that could affect medication choices

- Choose the best medication or combination of medications for the pain

Case studies

1. Mary Jones:

Mary Jones is a 45-year-old telephone operator who tells you her pain is at the level of 5/10 and that she has been taking 20 extra-strength Tylenol per day (500 mg per tablet) to control her upper back and neck pain. She says she has a prescription for a stronger pain medication, but is saving it for the stronger pain. What should you tell Mary about her pain management medications?

- Mary is exceeding the maximum daily dose of Tylenol.

- Moderate-level pain requires a combination opioid or opioid with or without an adjuvant.

- Medications that would be helpful for Mary are Vicodin-level medications, or Ultram, and a topical analgesic balm. If she begins to take the pain medication regularly, an extended-release medication such as oxycontin or Ultram ER would be helpful.

2. Susan Peters:

Susan Peters is a 35-year-old single mother who has been complaining of multiple sites of achiness at a moderate 6/10 pain intensity. She has seen many physicians and has been told she needs to see a psychologist to help her cope, since she under so much stress with her job as a waitress and caring for her children. Susan can't sleep well at night and says she feels tired all the time. Eventually, one of her physicians diagnoses her with fibromyalgia. What types of pain medications should Susan take for her pain? Since her pain is at the moderate level, should she be taking opioids?

- The APS Fibromyalgia (2005) Guidelines indicate that the medication of choice for fibromyalgia is amitriptyline and cyclobenzaprine (Flexeril), a muscle relaxant

- Ultram is also indicated in the practice guidelines for unrelieved pain

- Opioids should be avoided because they are only partially effective for this pain complaint and dose escalations are common since the pain continues at higher levels

3. Sam Waters:

Sam is your 75-year-old neighbor. He has always been active with gardening and walking around town. You haven't seen him for several days and go over to his house to check on him. He answers the door and tells you he has such pain in his knees that he can't stand it. He rates his pain as 6/10. You suggest he see his physician, which he does. The physician tells Sam that his osteoarthritis has worsened. Sam has a history of a heart attack—two years ago—and is on coumadin. What types of pain medication should Sam take for his arthritis pain?

- Sam should not take NSAIDs due to his history of heart attack and coumadin use.

- Sam should try Ultram to see whether it is effective for his pain. If the medication works well for him and he takes it regularly, Ultram ER would then be a good choice since the pain is constant over 24 hours.

- Another option for Sam's pain would be any moderate pain medication, such as Vicodin or Percocet.

- If Sam's pain is not relieved with these less-potent pain medications, he may need a Duragesic patch or another stronger, extended-release medication such as Oxycontin.

4. John Stone:

John is a 62-year-old man who has had diabetes for 20 years. His blood sugars are under control, he follows the recommended diabetic diet, and he exercises regularly. However, he has painful numbness in his feet that makes walking difficult. When you ask him to rate his pain, he tells you it is almost always a 5/10 level pain. The pain is worse at night. What medication can John use to help control his pain?

- John has neuropathy and requires a neuropathic pain medication

- Cymbalta is indicated for diabetic neuropathy and is well-tolerated if dosing is started low and escalated slowly

- TCAs would not be a good choice since John is an older adult

- He may also benefit from applying a lidoderm to the painful area or using a mild opioid

Practice exercises

Access the FDA Web site and review the information on NSAIDs. Review the patient education sheet to see what types of patient education the FDA recommends for patients who are taking these medications.

Non-pharmacologic pain management therapies

Learning objectives

After reading this chapter, the participant should be able to

- describe how cognitive behavioral techniques can be added to a pain management regimen

- discuss the use of non-pharmacologic therapies

Complementary and alternative medicine (CAM)

Recently there has been a great deal of discussion about complementary and alternative therapies for pain management. As a result of this discussion, the National Institutes of Health (NIH) has developed a National Center for Complementary and Alternative Medicine (NCCAM). The center's strategic plan for 2005–2009 hopes to develop a scientific basis for many therapies that are now being used without evidence-based support.

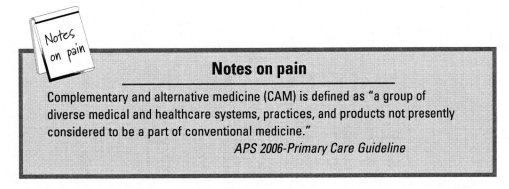

Notes on pain

Complementary and alternative medicine (CAM) is defined as "a group of diverse medical and healthcare systems, practices, and products not presently considered to be a part of conventional medicine."
APS 2006-Primary Care Guideline

Complementary and alternative therapies can be described as

- manipulative and body-based practices that include massage, heat, cold, and acupuncture

- cognitive behavioral approaches or mind-body work, such as relaxation, biofeedback, and imagery

- energy medicine, including Reiki and therapeutic touch (TT)

- nutritional approaches that incorporate the use of herbs and vitamin supplements

There have been many terms applied to non-pharmacologic therapies for pain relief. Here are some of the differences between the terms.

Notes on pain

Complementary: Techniques or additional therapies that are used in conjunction with recognized mainstream medical practices. For example, when acupuncture is used concurrently with medication for low back pain.

Alternative: This term means forgoing recognized medical therapy and using other treatments for a condition. For example, when vitamin supplements and imagery are used in place of radiation or chemotherapy for cancer treatment.

Integrative: A term coined by CAM practitioners to indicate the combined use of pharmacotherapy and non-pharmacologic methods for medical treatment. This term was popularized by Dr. Andrew Weil (O'Hara 2003).

Most Americans are open to using non-pharmacologic treatments for pain relief. Many have old home remedies that they often use for minor aches or pains. In a 1997 survey, Americans reported that they made 629 million visits to CAM practitioners (Eisenberg, D in Iyer 2003). In Europe and Australia, about 20% to 70% of all patients use CAM therapies (O'Hara 2003).

Despite the common usage of CAM therapies, there is still dissonance between CAM and recognized medical practice. Although 40% of patients discuss their use of CAM therapy with their primary care practitioner, many volunteer the information rather than respond to questions on the topic from physicians (O'Hara in Iyer, 2003). The following review of therapies will focus on the most common techniques used by patients.

Manipulative and body-based therapies

Heat and cold

Most patients will use heat and cold for pain relief at home even before they seek medical attention for a painful condition such as low back pain. Heat is used to decrease stiffness, reduce pain, and relieve muscle spasms (ASPMN 2002). Heat can be applied in many ways, such as with heat lamps, hot packs, or heating pads. Patients should be cautioned to use heat for short periods of time to avoid burning; to avoid using heat over mentholated analgesic balms, which increases the potential for skin damage; and to never place heating pads over analgesic patches such as Duragesic (Fentanyl), since the heat causes the medication to infuse more quickly and overdose may result.

Cold applications work by causing decreased nerve conduction, cutaneous counter irritation, vasoconstriction, muscle relaxation, and the reduction of local and systemic metabolic activity (ASPMN 2002). Cold therapy is indicated for muscle aches and sprains, muscle spasm, and contusions (ASPMN 2002). Cold therapies can be applied as ice baths, ice packs, or as ice massage. Patients should be cautioned about leaving the ice packs on too long, which can cause skin damage. Patients with decreased sensitivity, such as diabetics, should be cautioned about placing the packs over desensitized skin.

A Cochrane report for using heat or cold in low back pain patients has found the therapy to have limited support (French 2006). However, there is moderate evidence for using a heat wrap to reduce pain and increase functionality in this patient population (French 2006). RICE therapy (Rest, Ice, Compression, and Elevation) has been used successfully for treating minor injuries (Berry et al 2006).

Acupuncture

Acupuncture is one of the oldest CAM therapies. It was originally used by the Chinese to balance the yin and yang life forces (also known as Qi, the life force and blood), where imbalance was thought to create disease (O'Hara 2003, ASPMN 2002). When acupuncture is used to treat pain, thin needles are inserted through the skin at certain anatomical points (acupuncture points) that are thought to possess electrical properties (NCCAM 2004, Dillard 2005, ASPMN 2002). Once the needles are in place, they are manipulated by hand or electrically stimulated. This is thought to release neurotransmitters helpful to pain relief (Dillard 2005).

Acupuncture is the CAM modality that has been studied the most and has received the most support. Patient populations thought to benefit from acupuncture are cancer patients, facial and dental pain patients, and patients who experience labor pain, knee osteoarthritis, and fibromyalgia symptoms (Dillard 2005, APS 2005).

Massage

A Cochrane review of massage for low back pain patients found that this technique might be beneficial for pain relief in this population (Furlan 2006). Massage is well-accepted by patients. The NIH NCCAM defines massage as pressing, rubbing, and otherwise manipulating muscles and soft tissue in the body (NCCAM 2005). Some massage therapists use scented oils, such as lavender, or other compounds that are thought to further relax the body. The effect of massage is thought to be the relaxation and lengthening of muscles, which allows oxygen and increased blood flow into the affected area (NCCAM 2005).

Other forms of body-based therapies are chiropractic, magnet, and copper bracelet therapies. Although they may have a popular base, there is little research support at this time to confirm their use in current practice.

Cognitive behavioral therapy (CBT)

Relaxation

Relaxation is one of the most common non-pharmacologic therapies recommended for a variety of painful conditions. It has been found to be helpful for pain relief (Cole & Brunk 1999). Relaxation techniques result in the reduction of physical tension and the promotion of emotional well-being (NCCAM 2005). Relaxation techniques can be simple, such as regulating breathing, or more complex, such as using formalized relaxation tapes. The effect of relaxation is to reduce muscle tension and promote muscle relaxation (ASPMN 2002). Patients who reported benefit from using relaxation were those having surgical procedures, cancer patients, and chronic pain patients (Dillard 2005). Patients who use this technique report an improved sense of well-being and score higher in quality of life scales (Dillard 2005).

Imagery

Imagery is a technique whereby patients use a set of images to create a sense of control and relaxation. The technique encourages the patient to imagine a place he or she finds comfortable or soothing. The patient is encouraged to feel the place, smell it, taste it, and enjoy the feeling of comfort that the scenario provides (ASPMN 2002).

Imagery is a form of relaxation using a mental image. Reinforcement of the helpful images can be provided by verbal prompting or a tape with recorded prompts. For example, a patient can be told "see a lovely yellow lemon. Feel the shape and texture of the lemon in your hand. It is round, smooth, and very pleasing. Smell the lemon; the fragrance fills the room. Taste the tart sweetness of the lemon, all the while remembering the shape and feel of the lemon's smooth skin." This type of relaxation technique using an image is difficult for some patients, and some patients may have difficulty retaining the image or creating the scenario.

Other forms of cognitive behavioral therapy are hypnosis, biofeedback, and meditation. The use of these therapies has been practiced for many years in many cultures. All have support for use as complementary techniques that can help relieve pain (O'Hara 2003).

Energy medicine

Reiki

Reiki is a form of energy medicine that has been used in Eastern cultures to soothe both the mind and body. In this technique, a Reiki practitioner transmits energy either long distance or by directly placing hands on the patients (NCCAM 2005).

The Reiki practitioner places his or her hands on specific energy points, or chakras, on the recipient's body. By concentrating and trying to allow the flow of energy through any blocked points, the patients receive physical and emotional healing. Reiki should be practiced only after one receives training as one of the three levels of practitioners by a Reiki Master.

Therapeutic touch

Therapeutic touch (TT) is another form of energy therapy. However, despite its name, the practitioner does not touch the patient receiving the therapy. It is often mistakenly referred to as "laying on of hands." The premise of TT is that the practitioner's healing force transfers or channels energy, thereby positively affecting the recovery of the patient (NCCAM 2005). When the practitioner passes his or her hands over the patient, the healing forces put the patient's body into harmony, thus promoting healing and pain relief.

Both TT and Reiki require a practitioner who is trained to perform the maneuvers. As with any therapy, the success of the technique is at least partly dependent on the skills of the practitioner and the ability of patients to accept the type of therapy being offered. NCCAM is undertaking the study of energy therapies by creating a research format where controlled studies are possible.

Nutritional approaches

Nutritional supplements, such as vitamins or herbs, have long been used as folk remedies. In China, many people use herbs formulated as teas, capsules, extracts, or tablets for pain treatment (Dillard 2005). One frequently used herb, Corydalis, is an alkaloid with potent analgesic properties (Dillard 2005). It traditionally has been used for menstrual pain. Some Chinese herbal medicines have anticoagulant properties, which limit their use.

The biggest problem with herbal supplements is the lack of formal regulatory processes, whereas dietary supplements are categorized under the FDA's Dietary Supplement Health and Education Act of 1994, which requires quality, safety, and efficacy standards. Before using herbs and dietary supplements, patients should discuss these substances with their physician to ensure safety and carefully examine the listed ingredients and inspect the containers for certification of authenticity. As always, patients who are pregnant should be extremely careful when using a substance that does not have quality control measures or a safety profile.

Practice exercises

1. Learn more about a CAM modality that interests you. Go online and search for Reiki or relaxation. You can also go to the NIH Web site at *www.nih.gov* and search for "CAM" to find more information on these modalities and the NCCAM studies that are in progress.

Case Study: Susan Johnson

Susan is a 72-year-old patient who has osteoarthritis. She has been taking opioids for pain relief, but really does not like the way they make her feel. She says, "That fuzzy feeling is awful. I sleep all day and all night too. I need something different for my pain."

When you interview Susan, she tells you her pain is 5/10. She can't sleep well without "painkillers," she has decreased her activities to a bare minimum, she sends her husband to the grocery store, and she can't stand walking. She wants better pain relief, but does not want to take opioids.

A. What types of medication would be a better fit for Susan?

Acetaminophen around the clock or NSAIDs if she is a good candidate.

B. What types of CAM therapies would be helpful for Susan?

Heat, cold, massage, relaxation, Reiki. Herbal medications and nutritional supplements would not be effective for pain relief.

C. What patient education can you provide for Susan?

If Susan is open to alternative therapy ideas, the nurse could suggest Reiki or TT, but she needs to be open to the idea to be receptive. She could easily use heat and cold with proper patient education. Massage would be helpful. Relaxation tapes would be beneficial, but Susan would need training to use imagery. You can visit patient education Web sites—such as WebMD—to find handouts for Susan on these modalities.

Acute pain management

Learning objectives

After reading this chapter, the participant should be able to

- explain the safe implementation of patient controlled analgesia

- explain the key concepts of epidural analgesia

- discuss the role of regional analgesia techniques in acute pain management

Acute pain is pain that results from tissue injury, such as a musculoskeletal injury or surgical pain. This type of pain alerts the body to the fact that it has been injured. Berry et al (2006) define it as a "complex, unpleasant experience with emotional and cognitive as well as sensory features that occur in response to tissue trauma." Acute pain is not expected to last long, and it resolves within the normal healing period.

The Joint Commission standards for pain management define the usual expectations for pain management:

- Every patient has the right to have their pain assessed and reassessed regularly

- Patients have the right to adequate treatment for their pain

- There should be no barrier to pain management (language, for example)

- The patient should be involved in his or her pain management plan of care and receive education about pain management

- Pain should not interfere with rehabilitation

- A multidisciplinary group should develop policies and procedures for pain management and monitor outcomes

(JCAHO 2001)

Undertreatment of acute pain

Acute pain has consistently been reported as undertreated, according to the studies conducted in the 1980s by Marks & Sachar that identified the issue through the current time (Apfelbaum 2003). With the many types of medications, techniques, and modalities available to treat pain, it is difficult to understand just why acute pain remains problematic. However, one study of hospitalized patients in the 1990s found 61% of the 217 patients reported pain ratings of 7 to 10 within the last 24 hours (Berry et al 2006). Apfelbuam, reports that 73 million surgeries are performed annually in the United States, with 75% of the patients reporting pain after surgery (2003). Of those patients, 86% reported pain levels of extreme, severe pain to moderate pain.

If acute pain is not treated effectively, the result may be the development of a chronic pain condition. Syndromes like this are much more difficult to treat and have a negative impact on quality of life (D'Arcy 2007). Untreated pain can also adversely affect immune function (Page 2005).

Treating acute pain

Patients with minor acute pain—for example, an ankle sprain—may just need oral pain medication, some physical therapy, and rest. Oral medication for minor pain, such as acetaminophen and NSAIDs, were described in Chapter 5.

For surgical patients experiencing more severe pain, there are options for using IV medications that can provide patients with highly effective pain relief. PCA and epidural analgesia can help surgery patients mobilize faster and be more satisfied with their pain control (AHCPR 1992).

National guidelines for acute pain suggest aggressive treatment for acute pain (APS 2003), and many encourage a multimodal approach (Berry et al 2006).

Patient controlled analgesia

One of the most common methods for pain control after surgery is PCA. The concept was developed in the 1970s to help patients achieve more consistent pain relief and increase satisfaction with postoperative pain relief.

A PCA consists of a machine with a computerized pump that can be programmed to deliver various types of pain medication. The healthcare provider who orders the PCA determines the drug, dose, lockout, and 1- or 4-hour limit that should be programmed into the pump by the nurse.

Patients push a button to activate the pump. If a dose of medication is available to patients, the pump delivers a dose. The machine is preset to ensure that patients have access only to the amount of medication that the program allows.

Settings and medication choices for PCA use are outlined here:

- Typical medications for PCA use are morphine, hydromorphone (Dilaudid), and fentanyl.

- Usual starting doses are 1 milligram for morphine, 0.2 milligrams for Dilaudid, and 10 micrograms for fentanyl.

- Typical dose intervals are 6 or 8 minutes.

- Hospitals can choose between 1- and 4-hour limits. One-hour limits are becoming more common than the four-hour limits because the shorter time period allows the nurse to monitor usage sooner and adjust the PCA dose upward or downward as needed.

- Monitoring the number of times patients push the button to attempt to get a dose and actual injections can give the nurse an idea of the efficacy of the PCA. If the patient has significantly more attempts on the PCA than actual injections, it indicates the patient is working very hard to get pain relief and the dose may need to be adjusted. Alternatively, the patient may not understand how to use the PCA and may need education on how it works.

Patient benefits

Patients who are using PCA as a means of pain control are usually very satisfied with their postoperative pain control. National guidelines, such as the Agency for Health Care Policy and Research (AHCPR) Acute Pain Guideline in 1992, promoted the use of PCAs after finding that many patients preferred the PCA to intermittent injection (AHCPR 1992). The American Society of Anesthesiologists (ASA) recommends using PCA for postoperative pain relief, and the American Society of Postanesthesia Nurses (ASPAN) also supports the use of PCAs.

Intramuscular injections (IM) are no longer recommended for pain relief, because of irregular absorption of medication (APS 2003). Instead, the IV route, including PCA, is the preferred method for administering pain medication to patients with acute postoperative pain.

The ASPMN finds that there are specific advantages to using the PCA over intermittent injections of pain medication:

- Improved pain relief

- Patient has more control over pain relief

- Coughing and deep breathing is easier for the patient, and ambulation is facilitated

- Patient can maintain a steady opioid serum level and avoid the peaks and valleys of IM or intermittent opioid administration

- PCA can shorten hospital stay after major surgery

(ASPMN 2002)

PCA use

For the PCA to work efficiently, patients must receive enough medication as a loading dose to be comfortable. They can then maintain comfort using the PCA button to administer additional medication as needed.

When dealing with patients using PCAs, they should be encouraged to give themselves a dose of pain medication prior to activity to help them move more easily. Once the patient is able to take a diet, oral pain medication should be ordered and the patient should be transitioned from the PCA to an oral medication regimen.

Safety concerns

Within the last few years, there have been some concerns about the safety of PCA pumps. There have been several reported cases of overdose and death of a patient while on a PCA, and in each case the PCA has been directly linked to the event (ISMP 2003, JCAHO 2005, Bezyack 2006).

One of the primary causes of adverse events was programming errors by nurses. In one study examining PCA-related errors, 71% were related to misprogramming of the PCA pump, resulting in over- or underdosing the patient; 15% were related to human factors, resulting in the administration of the wrong medication; and 9% were related to equipment problems (Weir 2005).

Programming errors have been found to include

- confusion over milliliter versus milligram

- PCA bolus dose that is intended to be activated by the patient as needed was confused with a basal dose

- loading dose programmed where the basal dose should have been entered

- wrong lockout setting selected

- wrong medication concentration selected

(ISMP 2003)

Because of these errors, the Institute for Safe Medication Practices (ISMP) has made recommendations that can enhance safety:

- Two independent nurse checks of the PCA rate, medication concentration, and dose settings

- Identification of the IV line where the PCA is infusing

- Use of prefilled medication syringes or bags

- Use of standardized order set

Documentation of PCA use should be done at least every four hours, and the totals should be cleared and entered on a standard documentation sheet. Monitoring sedation levels should be a part of all PCA monitoring for nurses, since it is a sensitive indicator when respiratory depression occurs (Pasero & McCaffery 2002). Even patients who are experiencing significant oversedation can be roused to a higher level of consciousness and an increased respiratory rate (Cohen & Smetzer 2005).

Patients should be monitored every hour or two during the initial phase of PCA therapy to provide adequate assessment. Less intensive monitoring can be used for the remainder of the therapy time.

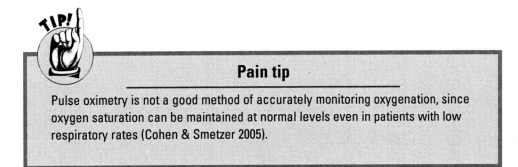

Pain tip

Pulse oximetry is not a good method of accurately monitoring oxygenation, since oxygen saturation can be maintained at normal levels even in patients with low respiratory rates (Cohen & Smetzer 2005).

Clinical practice issues

Two clinical practices related to safety issues with PCA use are the continuous infusion option for opioid naïve patients and PCA by proxy. The use of continuous infusions where the patient gets a small amount of opioid medication every hour is no longer encouraged, since it does little to contribute to analgesia and has the potential for oversedation (APS 2003, Acute Pain Management: Scientific Evidence 2005).

PCA by proxy—where someone other than the patient pushes the button for the patient—has serious consequences. No one but the patient can tell how sedated he or she is getting. If the patient does become sedated, he or she stops pushing the button, which has always been considered the built-in safety mechanism for the PCA.

PCA by proxy has been controversial for many years. There are documented cases of well-intentioned family members pushing the PCA button for oversedated patients, resulting in significant oversedation and, in some cases, death (Bezyack 2006, JCAHO 2005, ASPMN 2002).

To counteract this, some institutions place tags on the PCA buttons stating "only the patient to push PCA button." Other institutions provide patients with education instructing only the patient to activate the PCA button.

A new position statement by ASPMN indicates that using nurse-activated PCA may be an acceptable alternative to counteract these safety issues, but there is a special form and set of orders that should be used with this option. Information on this form of PCA can be accessed at *www.aspmn.org*.

The Joint Commission recommendations

The Joint Commission recommends these key elements to maintain the safety of patients using PCA pumps for self-delivery of pain medications:

- Select patients for PCA carefully. Patients who are cognitively impaired, confused, have sleep apnea, or are obese are not good candidates for PCA use. Infants also are unsuitable candidates for PCA.

- Monitor patients closely. Nurses need to know the difference between oversedation and other complications, such as pulmonary embolus or stroke, signs of opioid toxicity, and withdrawal.

- Teach patients and family members about the dangers of PCA by proxy: A sedated patient will not press the button to deliver opioid, thus avoiding toxicity.

- Place warning signs on all PCA pumps: "For patient use only."

- Ensure that PCA pumps are programmed correctly. Nurses should be taught how to program pumps correctly and maintain competency on PCA pumps, and their ability to enter a prescription should be validated.

(JCAHO 2005)

Epidural analgesia

Epidural analgesia is recommended for postoperative pain relief by the ASA 2004, the APS 2003, and the AHCPR 1992. Epidural analgesia involves inserting a thin plastic catheter into the epidural space in the perioperative time period. The epidural space is located just inside the vertebrae of the spine and is highly vascular, having a flat shape like a closed paper bag. As the anesthesiologist inserts an epidural needle into the epidural space, preservative-free normal saline is used to expand the space. The placement of the catheter is determined by the dermatome where the surgery and surgical incision will be located.

Expected levels for catheters would be

- high thoracic placement used for chest surgeries, such as a thoracotomy

- low thoracic placement for abdominal surgeries, such as an abdominal aortic aneurysm repair

- lumbar placement for surgeries on the lower extremities, such as a total knee replacements

Epidurals can also be placed for thoracic trauma to control pain. For patients with flail chest resulting from a fall or motor vehicle accident, an epidural catheter can provide excellent pain relief, allowing earlier mobilization and facilitating respiratory efforts. The only limitation for epidural catheter placement is the patient physiology, such as damage to the patient's spine from past surgeries or congenital malformations, and changes related to chronic conditions such as arthritis.

Medication choices

The two medications recommended by the ASA for use in epidural catheters are morphine and fentanyl (ASA 2004). Dilaudid and sufentanil have less evidence for use. The benefit to epidural catheters is the ability to combine a local anesthetic—such as bupivacaine or ropivacaine—in an epidural solution. This combination of medications can provide excellent pain relief, and the concentration of the local anesthetic is usually low enough to allow patients to ambulate. All medications used in epidural analgesia must be preservative-free, since many medication preservatives are neurotoxic.

Patient care

Epidural analgesia is delivered using a pump similar to the PCA pump. Epidural pain relief usually involves a low continuous rate such as 6 to 8 milliliters an hour, with a patient controlled epidural analgesia (PCEA) dose that can be delivered in the same way as a PCA bolus dose: upon pushing a button to activate a bolus dose from the preprogrammed epidural pump. Careful monitoring is required because the patient has control of medication delivery.

Caring for patients with epidural analgesia in the postoperative period requires regular monitoring and evaluation. Postoperative monitoring should be done at least every 2–4 hours after the initial postoperative period. Nurses should work with patients who are using epidural analgesia in order to get the information needed for a complete assessment.

Key elements of an epidural assessment include

- pain intensity rating.

- oxygen saturation.

Pain Management: Evidence-Based Tools and Techniques for Nursing Professionals

- type of medication infusing, concentration, dose, epidural pump settings, attempts and injections, secure connectors.

- observation of the integrity of the epidural insertion site, including any signs of leakage, errythema, swelling, or drainage. The dressing should be intact at all times.

- assessment of epidural tubing, which should be clearly marked "for epidural use only," to avoid connecting any other type of fluid or medication to the epidural line.

- regular assessment of side effects, such as pruritis, nausea/vomiting, and any paresthesia or motor block.

Treat pruritis and nausea with the medications that are ordered. To assess for temporary paresthesia or motor block, patients should be instructed to push their buttocks up from the bed. Looking for quadriceps strength is very important. If patients can lift themselves from the bed, they should be able to bear weight when asked to ambulate. Turning the epidural rate down or changing the local anesthetic solution can help resolve the paresthesia/motor block. No patient should be asked to get out of bed without an assessment for paresthesia or motor block.

Safety issues

Patients and family members should be educated about epidural analgesia. As with the PCA, epidural by proxy is not recommended.

Most anticoagulants are problematic with epidural catheters because of the fear of epidural hematoma. If the patient's blood is too thin, tissue damage when the catheter is placed or removed can result in blood collection in the epidural space, resulting in spinal cord compression. If the clot is not promptly removed, permanent paraplegia can result. The ASRA recommendations for use of anticoagulants with regional anesthesia can be found at *www.asra.com*.

Regional analgesia techniques

Peripheral nerve blocks are now becoming some of the most common and successful adjunct techniques for pain relief. With this technique, a local anesthetic block is provided directly at the site of expected pain. Common blocks include intercostals, ilioinguinal, penile, plexus, or femoral blocks. Femoral blocks can be performed either as a single shot given during the immediate postoperative period or as a continuous infusion. Continuous nerve blocks can be provided with several types of systems, such as ON-Q (discussed in the next section.)

Regional anesthesia techniques can help patients mobilize more quickly. Reports are favorable, with many patients reporting high satisfaction with the techniques when they are combined with a standard postoperative pain measure, such as a PCA (Idelli 2005).

Comparing the use of morphine PCA and femoral nerve block, Singelyn (2005) found that total hip replacement patients reported similar pain relief with both techniques, but the patients with the femoral block reported fewer technical difficulties and fewer side effects. In another study, Liu (2003) found that patients were more satisfied with pain control and had earlier mobilization and fewer side effects when a peripheral nerve block was used for postoperative pain control.

Most pain management authorities recommend the use of multimodal pain management (ASA 2004, APS 2003, Berry et al 2006). Using a standard pain management technique and adding a regional technique can help patients achieve more satisfaction with their postoperative pain control, eliminate some side effects of medication management, and help patients mobilize earlier.

New techniques on the horizon

ON-Q

ON-Q is a local anesthetic delivery system that consists of a ball containing local anesthetic, which is attached to a catheter placed either directly on the femoral nerve, directly into a joint space such as a shoulder, or laced along a surgical incision. The catheter has multiple holes along the end, allowing for localized delivery of a local anesthetic such as bupivacaine. The ball reservoir is filled at the time of catheter placement and can be programmed for a set flow rate.

FIGURE 7.1	ON-Q

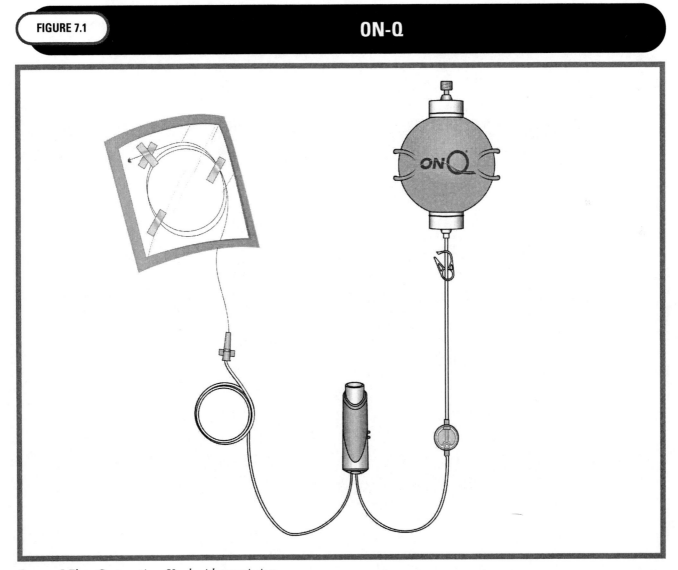

Source: I-Flow Corporation. Used with permission.

Depending on the rate selected, the reservoir should remain full for several days. The catheter can be removed either by a patient who has received education on catheter removal or by a healthcare provider (D'Arcy 2007).

The latest version of the system is called the ON-Q Bloc. It not only provides a continuous flow of local anesthetic, but has a button activation cord that the patient can use to deliver additional doses of local anesthetic when needed for increased pain or activity.

IONSYS

IONSYS is a new medication delivery system that uses fentanyl. The system is about the size of a credit card and is attached to the patient's upper arm. It requires no lines and does not use a pump. The patient can push a button to deliver medication via iontophoresis.

FIGURE 7.2 — **IONSYS**

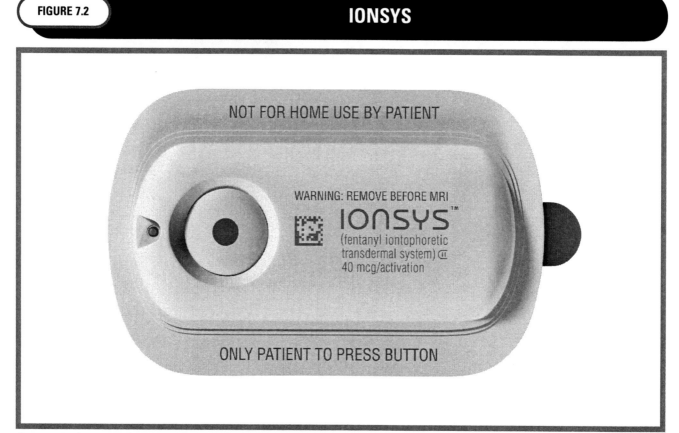

Source: Ortho-McNeil, Inc. Used with permission.

> ### Notes on pain
>
> **Iontophoresis:** A method of delivering medication by passing a mild electrical current across the skin to drive the medication into the dermis.

The IONSYS has a fentanyl reservoir that is preprogrammed to deliver a dose of 40 micrograms of fentanyl, up to six doses per hour and at ten-minute intervals (D'Arcy 2005; Viscusi 2004, 2005, and 2006; D'Arcy 2007). To activate the system, the patient pushes a button on the top of the device. The system continues until the maximum of 80 doses are delivered or after 24 hours, at which point the system stops. This system is designed to maintain pain control once the patient has reached an adequate level of pain control after surgery. At least two-thirds of the patients in a study group with IONSYS were very satisfied with the pain control the device provided (Viscusi 2006).

Key elements of managing acute pain

Acute pain management is challenging, but there are many options for controlling pain.

The key elements of acute pain management are

- aggressive pain management to intervene early to relieve elevated pain levels and prevent the development of harder-to-treat chronic pain syndromes, such as CRPS

- frequent assessment and reassessment of pain

- multimodal techniques for pain management

- safe use of PCA and PCEA for appropriate patients

- advanced pain management techniques, such as epidural analgesia and regional techniques for patients in need of a higher level of pain relief

- regular delivery of pain medication to avoid undertreating postoperative pain

---

Practice exercises

1. Access The Joint Commission Web site and the ISMP Web site and look at the recommendations for safety when using PCA.

Case Study: Carol Smith

Carol Smith is a 44-year-old female patient who is admitted to the surgical unit after an abdominal hysterectomy. She is using a morphine PCA for pain relief. She cannot take oral pain medication yet, as she is NPO. When you enter the room, she says, "I am so sick to my stomach. I just keep vomiting and vomiting. The pain control is awful. I haven't been able to get my pain under control all night."

When you look at the PCA, you see that she is using PCA morphine, which has a high profile for the side effect of nausea and vomiting. The PCA records she has made 115 attempts and received 20 injections. She hasn't pushed the button in the last 2 hours. Her pump is set at 1 milligram of morphine every 8 minutes. What can you do to improve her pain control?

Correct actions include:
   a. Administering regular doses of antiemetics to relieve the nausea.
   b. Changing the medication to another medication—such as Dilaudid—to hope for fewer side effects.
   c. Give loading doses of a new medication to get Carol comfortable.
   d. Convert to intermittent IV medication that will not control the pain as well as the PCA.

The fact that she has not pushed the button in the last 2 hours tells you she has no faith in the current pain regimen. You will have to make changes that will provide confidence.

Practice exercises (cont.)

Case Study: Peter Jones

Peter Jones, a 67-year-old man, has just had total joint replacement. For his postoperative pain control, he is using an epidural PCEA with fentanyl and bupivacaine. He calls you into his room the morning after his surgery and tells you, "I had my wife push the button for me a few times last night, and this morning I can't move my leg, and I just can't seem to stay awake. I don't have any pain, but I am worried that the numbness in my leg is permanent."

Peter has been ordered on coumadin for anticoagulant prophylaxis for DVT. What is happening to Peter? Does he have an epidural hematoma?

Rationale:

Peter has violated one of the primary rules for PCEA use: He had his wife push the button. This has resulted in paresthesia and mild oversedation. The appropriate actions are

- check O2 saturation and place him on oxygen if it is low
- stop the PCEA and notify anesthesia
- alert all staff that Peter has paresthesia and should not be taken out of bed until it resolves
- prepare to give Narcan, an opioid reversal agent, if Peter's oxygenation saturation level is low or his respiratory rate starts to slow below 8 per minute
- continue frequent monitoring
- restart the epidural at a reduced rate once the numbness resolves

The paresthesia will resolve slowly over a period of several hours. The PCEA can be turned off until the numbness resolves or pain returns. The medication delivery rate can be lowered if needed, or the solution can be changed if numbness persists to a lesser degree.

Practice exercises (cont.)

Coumadin takes from 24 to 48 hours to become fully active. If Peter is dosed at a rate to keep the INR (the measure of blood thinness used for coumadin) at 1.5 or lower, the recommended ASRA tolerance level for patients on coumadin and epidural analgesia, Peter should be fine. He most likely does not have a hematoma, since he is only postop day 1 and his first dose of coumadin was less than 24 hours prior to the event.

One of the basic elements of epidural safety was violated here. Peter and his wife will need to be educated on how to use the PCEA appropriately. Peter is the only one who should push the PCEA button, and his wife should not continue to push the button for Peter.

Chronic pain management

Learning objectives

After reading this chapter, the participant should be able to

- identify interventional therapies used to treat chronic pain

Reasons for chronic pain

Chronic pain is very common today. It can stem from a variety of sources:

- Low back pain as the result of trauma, failed back surgery, or chronic diseases such as degenerative disc disease or arthritis

- Chronic illness, such as rheumatoid arthritis, osteoarthritis, multiple sclerosis, or peripheral vascular disease

- Neuropathic conditions, such as diabetic neuropathy, postherpetic neuralgia, or complex regional pain syndrome

- Conditions that occur as the result of treatment, such as post mastectomy or post thoracotomy pain, post chemotherapy–related neuropathies, or nerve entrapment syndromes resulting from surgery, such as post hysterectomy pain syndrome

Chronic pain does not respect any person and can occur without any sign of physical damage. Some patients say, "I just got up with the pain," and cannot point to a specific cause. Chronic or persistent pain is pain that lasts beyond the normal healing period and is present for at least six months. It can be present without any signs of physical damage (D'Arcy 2005). Patients with chronic pain experience their pain at varying degrees throughout the day and night.

The cost of pain

The cost of chronic pain is immense. Approximately 40% of the American population experiences chronic pain, with higher percentages in nursing homes (Roper Starch 2001, Gibson & Bol 2001). The best estimate of monetary loss related to lost worker productivity is $61 billion per year (Stewart et al 2003). If lost income and medical expenses are added to the lost productivity costs, the total figure for economic impact rises to $100 billion per year.

At a more personal level, Professor John Liebeskind at the University of California has determined that chronic pain can kill by suppressing the immune response. As chronic pain suppresses the natural killer cells, the body loses its ability to defend itself against some types of tumor cells and virus-infected cells (D'Arcy 2006).

The perception of chronic pain

As the body feels pain (**nociception**), it determines there has been an injury and responds naturally. With continued nociception, the body changes the way it perceives the pain stimulus. Neural pathways become hypersensitive to the repeated pain stimuli, and n-methyl-d-aspartate (NMDA) receptors are activated. The purpose of these NMDA receptors is to promote the pain stimulus and help it transmit more quickly and with more intensity (Dubner 2005).

As the nerves carrying the pain stimulus continue to be activated, the central nervous system becomes highly excited and sensitized to pain as pain-facilitating neurotransmitters such as substance P and bradykinin are continuously released. The secondary effect as the pain stimulus continues is secondary hyperalgesia, where even a slightly painful sensation is perceived as extremely painful (Dubner 2005).

If the pain is the result of a nerve injury, it is classed as neuropathic. Some neuropathic syndromes include phantom limb pain, post mastectomy pain syndrome, postherpetic neuralgia, and diabetic neuropathy. In these conditions, the injured nerve cells tend to create a pain that patients identify as burning, "like a blow torch being fired on my chest," painful pins and needles, shooting, or shocklike (Staats et al 2004).

Pain tip

When assessing a patient with chronic pain, be sure to ask the quality of the pain sensation. Refer to the multidimensional assessment scales in Chapter 4 for more information. If the patient uses a verbal descriptor that indicates a neuropathic pain, such as burning or tingling, the medications used to treat the pain will be different: antiseizure medication, antidepressants, or topical applications of Lidoderm patches or capsaicin cream.

Differences between chronic and acute pain

Patients who are experiencing chronic pain are different from patients with acute pain. There may be no physiologic changes, such as increased blood pressure, and the patients may not outwardly appear as though they are in pain. Most chronic pain patients have learned to adapt and present a different appearance to the world—a social mask—that hides their true pain experiences.

Chronic pain patients may have difficulty telling you what their pain level is using a 0 to 10 pain intensity scale. Their pain ratings may be consistently higher despite changes in pain medications. Success with analgesic regimens may instead need to be judged on increased ability to function (Wilson et al 1997).

Depression is common in chronic pain patients. A complete pain assessment should include an assessment for depression and questions about a patient's mood. (See the multidimensional pain assessment tools in Chapter 4.) Studies have shown that chronic pain patients have twice the rate of suicide than people without pain (Tang & Crane 2006), so antidepressant therapy and a consult for assessment by a psychologist are clearly indicated for any patient who demonstrates signs of depression or suicidal ideation.

Sleep disturbances are also very common, and 55% of patients in one study reported restless/light sleep after the onset of pain (Marin et al 2006). This sleep deprivation only increases the physical toll that chronic pain takes on a patient.

Prevent chronic pain syndromes

Aggressive treatment of acute pain is indicated to prevent the development of difficult to treat chronic pain syndromes such as Complex Regional Pain Syndrome (CRPS). This syndrome is usually a result of an injury, trauma, or surgery where repeated activation of a pain stimulus creates central sensitization.

Patient with CRPS will demonstrate allodynia, thermal changes (heightened sensitivity to heat and cold), and changes in skin color and appearance (D'Arcy 2007). Nurses should be suspicious if patients with acute pain continue to complain of high levels of unrelieved pain. CRPS can be avoided if acute pain is treated early and aggressively, but once CRPS develops it is an extremely difficult syndrome to manage. A multimodal approach—with medications, physical therapy, topicals, and possibly a spinal cord stimulator—will be needed (Harden 2005).

Case study: Gene Rogers

Gene is an avid race car enthusiast. Last year he was driving more than 100 miles per hour when he crashed into the side rail of a raceway track. He had many injuries at the time of the accident, but most have healed. The one thing that is still painful is his left leg, which was amputated below the knee. He says the pain is always 6/10 and it aches all day and night. He tells a nurse: "If I knew then what I do now, I certainly would have been more cautious. This pain never goes away; I can't sleep and I have lost 25 pounds. I just have no appetite for anything. I get up in the morning and I am supposed to go to therapy. I can't work with the therapist because of the shooting pain that goes up my amputated leg when they move it and, strangely, I feel the pain in my amputated foot. Am I crazy to say I feel pain where there is no leg? I take my pain pills; why don't they help with the pain?"

Questions

1. Does Gene have chronic pain? If so what type?
Gene has phantom limb pain, which is chronic neuropathic pain. Phantom limb pain, felt by as many as 80% of all limb amputees, can be minimized with aggressive postoperative analgesia (Gevirtz 2005). The sensation of the amputated limb is common and may resolve over a period of months as neural pathways are rerouted.

2. What other symptoms of chronic pain does Gene have?
Depression, indicated by poor appetite, sleep disturbance

3. What types of therapies would be most helpful to Gene?
Opioid and neuropathic pain medications, such as antiseizure medications; antidepressants; and topical applications of local anesthetic (Lidoderm patches). Psychological support, physical therapy, grief counseling for inability to drive race cars.

Therapies for treating chronic pain

Medications and combinations of medications, such as opioids and antisiezure medications, are recommended for use in many chronic pain conditions, such as sickle cell disease, arthritis, and postherpetic neuralgia, (D'Arcy & McCarberg 2004, APS 2002, 2004, 2005). Remember that if the patient has consistent pain through the day, using an extended-release medication with adequate short-acting breakthrough medication may be the most helpful.

Most chronic pain patients will need a multimodal approach, with medications as only one part of the therapy. See Chapter 6 for a discussion of psychosocial/behavioral approaches and complementary therapies such as relaxation and imagery.

There may be indications that an intervention from a pain management specialist is appropriate. Most interventional pain management specialists are anesthesiologists, and the procedures and techniques are performed in an anesthesiology-based pain clinic.

Interventional options for treating chronic pain

Epidural steroid injections

Epidural steroid injections consist of injecting a steroid and local anesthetic into the epidural space directly adjacent to the nerve that is producing the pain. By placing the steroid solution directly at the site of pain generation, it is hoped that the pain and inflammatory process can be decreased. The local anesthetic provides immediate relief; the steroid can take up to 5–7 days to become fully active. This bimodal approach can be very helpful for reducing pain, but patients must be told about the delay in activation (Wilson et al 1997).

Patients are usually injected with the solution in a pain clinic where fluoroscopy can be used to locate the area of the pain-producing nerve. The patient is placed on a cart, and the fluoroscope is moved over the patient to locate the site for injection. The steroid and local anesthetic are injected into the nerve root after an additional local anesthetic is used to numb the skin. Patients may receive up to three injections per year. The ASA recommends a neurological workup prior to the injection, as well as a follow-up evaluation to monitor increased functionality, pain relief, and any adverse effects (Wilson et al 1997).

The following patients are good candidates for epidural, selective nerve root, or facet injections:

- Patients with low back pain with a radicular (pain radiating down the leg) component

- Patients where arthritis has narrowed the spinal facet and the nerves coming through the opening are being compressed

- Patients where a specific nerve is being impinged and compressed, creating pain in a specific dermatome

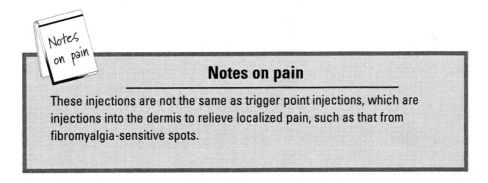

Notes on pain

These injections are not the same as trigger point injections, which are injections into the dermis to relieve localized pain, such as that from fibromyalgia-sensitive spots.

Implanted therapies

If a patient has increased his or her pain medication consumption to near the daily total maximum or has neuropathic pain, an implanted therapy such as an implanted morphine pump or a spinal cord stimulator may be indicated.

Intrathecal pumps

Intrathecal pumps are placed in a pocket of skin on the abdomen, usually below the beltline in the lower abdominal quadrant, along with a catheter that is tunneled around the body into the intrathecal space. The medication is placed into the pump reservoir with a thin needle that goes through the skin into the reservoir port.

There are several different producers for these implanted pumps, but the concept is the same for all: A computerized chip in the pump is programmed to deliver the medication intrathecally at a preset rate. The computer chip in the pump can be read by a handheld external programmer that identifies the patient, the medication in the pump, the delivery rate, and the date the pump should be refilled.

The two drugs that are approved for use in these pumps are preservative-free morphine and baclofen. Morphine is used for pain relief in patients who have escalated doses of different opioid pain medications without optimal pain relief. Intrathecal baclofen is used for patients with neurologic diseases such as multiple sclerosis, to reduce muscle rigidity in patients who have maximized the daily doses of oral baclofen.

The advantage of this system is that it delivers a small amount of pain medication and provides improved pain relief. The disadvantages are the need for dose titration, requiring return visits to the pain clinic for refills; the potential for catheter kinking or occlusion; and possible irritation in the spinal membranes, which causes scarring and can create granulomas (Staats & Wallace 2004). The patient also has no control over the pump rate, and changes can only be made by a physician using the computerized programmer.

Spinal cord stimulators

Another type of intervention designed to treat neuropathic pain is the spinal cord stimulator. For patients who have not responded to neuropathic pain medications and have tried a modality such as TENS (transcutaneous electrostimulation) unsuccessfully, spinal cord stimulation is a second-line option (Wilson 1997).

Spinal cord stimulators are placed while the patient is awake so that pain relief can be targeted to the specific nerves producing the pain. A set of catheters with electrodes at the tip are placed into the epidural space, and a mild electrical current is generated to the area where the pain is being produced.

Once the patient states they feel a tingling sensation in the painful area, the catheter is secured for a trial period. If the trial provides a reduction in pain, a permanent placement is done, with a small pacemaker-sized battery internalized (D'Arcy 2004). The sensation the patient feels is a tingling in the area of pain, not a full relief of painful sensation.

With the spinal cord stimulator, the healthcare provider has the ability to turn the various electrodes off and on and change the poles on individual leads. This changes the area that is being stimulated. The patient can turn the stimulator off and on using a small handheld device that communicates with the implanted battery. With this technique the patient has some control over the device. Disadvantages are battery failure, infection, lead breakage, or migration out of the area where the catheter was originally placed.

There are special considerations before using an implanted therapy for pain relief. Proper patient selection is key to the success of implanted modalities.

- Oral analgesia doses should have reached maximum doses with several different medications

- Intolerable side effects are experienced, despite opioid rotation

- Improved analgesia during trial of intrathecal or spinal cord stimulation

- Physiologic stability and realistic goals

- The patient accepts the need for the modality and is able to travel to a clinic for care and refills

- Intractable spasticity unrelieved by oral antispasmodics

(Staats & Wallace 2004)

Nurses who care for patients with implanted systems should be aware of what medications are in the intrathecal pump and the daily dose being delivered. This information can be obtained by an interrogation of the pump using the computerized programmer. Patients with implanted pumps may also use oral pain medication to supplement the pump and may need breakthrough medication for increased activity. These patients should also be monitored for any sign of infection, such as pain, increased white counts, or fever.

Spinal cord stimulator patients are most often able to report a change in stimulation pattern or a lack of power when the battery fails. Nurses should assess patients with both types of devices for pain relief and increases in functionality. Although these patients may report high pain intensity scores, they may also report being able to do activities that were too difficult prior to the implantation. Quality of life for these patients may not be based on reduction in pain but rather as increased functionality.

Radiofrequency ablation and epiduroscopy

Radiofrequency ablation and epiduroscopy are two of the newer interventions for chronic pain relief. Although theses techniques are not first-line options, they are being performed and some patients are finding pain relief (D'Arcy 2004).

With radiofrequency lesioning, a physician uses a heated probe to sever a sensory nerve branch that serves an area of the body that the patient has identified as painful. Although this technique is usually done for low back pain, in one study with patients who had hip pain, the pain intensity scores for the patients preprocedure were 6.8 but decreased to 2.7 post-lesioning (Kawaguchi 2001). The effect of the radiofrequency lesioning process can last for up to 18 months.

With epiduroscopy, a physician inserts a scope with a camera into the epidural space, and then scar tissue on nerve roots is located and removed using a laser or specifically adapted surgical tools (Ruetten 2002). To date, the video quality from the epiduroscope is less than optimal, and clinical reports indicate cloudy images and a low visual field. The technique also requires a physician who has been trained and has experience with the technique.

For some patients with chronic pain, epiduroscopy or radiofrequency lesioning has provided pain relief. Given the high number of patients who suffer from chronic pain and the huge impact that the pain has on everyday functioning, some patients who have failed other techniques and are candidates for these techniques are willing to try a new approach.

Practice exercises

---

1. Access one of the Web sites for chronic pain and find information on the condition or the devices that can be used for chronic pain relief.
   - Chronic pain association: *www.acpa.org*
   - Medtronic: *www.medtronic.com*
   - Cochrane reviews for chronic pain: *www.cochrane.org*

Case Study: Joan Johnson

Joan has been referred to a pain clinic for burning pain that radiates from her low back to her knee. She had back surgery twice in the past two years with little or no relief. She says it is so distressing she cannot continue with her daily activities or hobbies, and her husband has become very distant. She has tried multiple pain medications, but she has only a mild reduction in pain. She reports her pain level to be 8/10 at the worst and 5/10 at the very best. Her sleep is disturbed, and she sleeps in a different bedroom from her husband so she does not wake him at night. What can the physician offer Joan to help her pain?

A. What type of pain is Joan experiencing?
Chronic neuropathic pain.

B. What types of medication should Joan have tried before her pain clinic referral?
Opioids, antiseizure medication, antidepressants, and topicals, such as Lidoderm patches/capsaicin cream.

C. What are some signs of the effect of chronic pain in Joan's life?
Impaired functional ability, emotional distance from her husband, and sleep disturbances.

Practice exercises (cont.)

D. What type of modality/medication/interventions do you think the pain physician will offer Joan?

If the doses of medications for pain relief have not been maximized, Joan may be put on a trial of a combination of these medications at high doses. If medications at increased doses do not improve pain relief, Joan may be candidate for a spinal cord stimulator. She would need to have a trial lead placement; if that is successful, a permanent spinal cord stimulator would be placed.

Difficult to treat pain conditions and specialty populations

Learning objectives

After reading this chapter, the participant should be able to

- determine appropriate treatment options for patients with difficult to treat pain syndromes

- identify barriers to pain management in older patients

There are some pain conditions where providing pain relief is difficult at best. Patients with low back pain, fibromyalgia, and a history of substance abuse are several groups that most practitioners find complex. Some of these pain syndromes have been briefly discussed in earlier chapters, but this chapter provides more in-depth information and treatment options for these complicated pain syndromes and conditions.

Managing low back pain

Low back pain (LBP), one of the most common pain complaints, may be caused by any number of sources:

- Degenerative changes from arthritis, disc disease, facet disease, bone spurs

- Musculoskeletal stress and strain

- Structural damage to spinal processes

- Malignancy or infection

(D'Arcy 2006)

The back consists of the cervical, thoracic, lumbar, and caudal spinal levels. Each vertebra is supported and separated by a gelatinous disc filled with fluid that provides cushioning and flexibility. From each of the spinal processes come a variety of nerves that pass through the spinal facets (wing-like projections on each side of the spine). If injury, aging, or disease cause changes in the spinal anatomy, pain can result.

Patients with the following risk factors have the potential for developing low back pain (LBP):

- Poor physical condition and no regular exercise

- Over 55 years of age

- Workers who have engaged in hard physical labor over a period of time (e.g., construction workers)

- Obesity

- Reduced spinal canal dimensions and spinal stenosis

- Lower socioeconomic groups with less access to healthcare

(Dorsi in Staats & Wallace 2004, D'Arcy 2006)

In addition to these risk factors there are some red flags that should be assessed. If a patient complains of significant weight loss without intentionally trying to lose weight or has pain that worsens at night and does not resolve with rest, then healthcare providers should suspect a malignancy.

Neurologic symptoms such as bowel and bladder dysfunction or worsening foot drop can signal a spinal cord compression or a neurologic disease. A progressive weakening in the lower extremities may indicate a cauda equine syndrome. Acute LBP may be caused by kidney or urinary tract infection or gynecologic conditions such as cystic ovaries that can be treated with antibiotics or other medications.

Acute LBP is different from chronic LBP. Patients with acute LBP will have pain that resolves within 6 to 12 weeks, regardless of the treatment regimen (Hagen 2006). Patients who do not improve within that time frame—about 15% of cases—are considered to have chronic LBP (Von Korff 1996).

Treatment options for acute LBP include

- staying active; bed rest is no longer considered beneficial for acute low back pain

- analgesic balms, heat, ice, or massage

- a pain medication that fits the level of pain the patient is reporting (See Chapter 5)

- a short course of non-selective NSAIDs or a COX-2 medication if the patient is a good candidate

For chronic LBP, treatment options include

- physical therapy for strength and mobility training

- acupuncture, heat, ice, and analgesic balms

- analgesic medications and opioids (either short-acting if the pain is not present all day or extended-release opioids if the pain is present the entire day and night)

- antidepressants and sleep medication as needed

- referral to a chronic pain management program where coping skills and a positive image are reinforced

- a referral for an epidural steroid injection

Notes on pain

For more information on both acute and chronic low back pain, including reviews of treatment options, visit the Cochrane review Web site and search for "low back pain."

Case study: Mary Hammond

Mary Hammond is a 54-year-old patient who hurt her back moving a large piece of furniture in her new home. She has been trying to treat her pain at home using over-the-counter NSAIDs, an analgesic balm, and a heating pad. She originally went to see her physician, who told her that she had a herniated disc, but she was not a surgical candidate. She has been in bed for periods of time over the last eight months. Now she feels very depressed and hopeless, since the pain is not getting any better.

Diagnostically, a straight leg raise reproduces pain in her back. The pain does not radiate down her leg. When she went to the physician he gave her a pre-scription for Vicodin, which did help her pain, but he was reluctant to keep giving her pain medications. Mary is at a loss as to what to do for her pain. She cannot finish decorating her new home, and she cannot keep treating the pain at home. She says the pain is at least a 5/10 on most days. What options does Mary have for her low back pain?

Questions
1. Should Mary continue on opioids?
Mary may need opioids at some times, but at others she may not. If Mary is a good candidate, using an NSAID might be a non-opioid option. Muscle relaxants and opioids may be the best treatment plan for flare ups.

2. Should Mary try other doctors to see whether they will perform surgery?
Mary has had a full diagnostic workup that indicates she has a herniated disc. At this time she is not a surgical candidate. Since she has had a comprehensive workup for her pain, it is highly unlikely that another doctor would decide on surgery. If Mary sees several other doctors, she may be accused of "doctor shopping." Requesting a second opinion from another physician may be the best approach.

3. What options would you suggest to Mary to treat her chronic low back pain?
Treatment options for Mary's chronic LBP include physical therapy for strength-ening and mobility, NSAIDs if she is a good candidate with no cardiovascular risks, opioids for flares, antidepressants and a medication for sleep if needed, heat, ice, acupuncture, or a referral to a pain clinic for an epidural steroid injec-tion. Lumbar supports are one therapy that has not been found to help chronic low back pain (Van Tulder 2004).

Pain management for fibromyalgia patients

Fibromyalgia is considered to be a diagnosis of exclusion. Nonetheless, it is still a very debilitating chronic pain syndrome and one that is extremely difficult to treat. There are no laboratory tests that can be used to confirm diagnosis, so subjective data must be used to determine a diagnosis. Since diagnosis is so difficult, patients often suffer debilitating pain for years before the cause of the pain is confirmed.

Patients with fibromyalgia have these characteristics in common:

• Painful tender points at multiple sites on the body

• Sleep disturbance

• Fatigue

• Mood disturbances

(Goldenberg 2004, D'Arcy & McCarberg 2006, APS 2005)

Less frequent complaints include

• cognitive loss

• irritable bowel or bladder

• restless legs

• temporomandibular joint pain

• anxiety, depression, or panic attacks

(APS 2005, D'Arcy & McCarberg 2006)

 Pain Management: Evidence-Based Tools and Techniques for Nursing Professionals

Fibromyalgia occurs in 2–5% of the United States population. The majority of patients diagnosed with fibromyalgia are women (3.5–7%), while only 0.5–2% are men (Goldenberg 2004). Many patients who have complaints of pain that could be diagnosed as fibromylagia are told "it is all in your head" and referred to psychologists.

There are, however, some specific criteria that are used to help in diagnosing the condition:

- Widespread bilateral pain above and below the waist of at least three months duration

- Excessive tenderness on applying pressure to 11 of 18 muscle-tendon sites ("tender points")

(Wolfe 1990)

Five independent studies have found that fibromyalgia patients have three to five times the normal amount of substance P in the cerebrospinal fluid (Goldenberg 2004). Additionally, nerve growth factor levels are also elevated, which is thought to affect sensory processing (Wolfe 1990). Deficits of serotonin, norepinephrine, and dopamine have also been found, suggesting a connection between fibromyalgia and some types of depressive syndromes (D'Arcy & McCarberg 2006).

The APS's fibromylagia pain treatment guidelines can be found on the Web site at *www.ampainsoc.org*. Recommendations for treating fibromylagia include the following:

- Amitriptyline (Elavil)

- Cyclobenzaprine (Flexeril)

- Cardiovascular exercise

- Cognitive behavioral therapy (CBT)

- Patient education

- Multidisciplinary therapy, such as exercise and CBT

Other treatment options with modest evidence for support include strength training, acupuncture, biofeedback, tramadol, SSRIs, SNRIs, and pregabelin. Therapies with weak evidence for support include massage therapy, ultrasound, chiropractic, SAMe, 5-HTP, and growth hormone. Treatments that have no evidence for support include trigger point injections, nutritional herbal remedies, opioids, corticosteroids, NSAIDs, benzodiazepines, calcitonin, melatonin, guaifenesin, and DHEA (APS 2005).

The saddest part of working with the diagnosis of fibromayalgia is the lack of acceptance in the medical community. Patients are often dismissed from primary care providers to psychiatric clinics. Nurses should be aware of not only the disease process of fibromyalgia, but also the emotional and psychological components that accompany the syndrome. A care plan aimed at helping a patient with fibromyalgia should include support for body image and a referral to a fibromyalgia support group.

> ## Case study: Jane Simmons
>
> Jane is a 42-year-old single mother who works as a waitress in a downtown café. She is having difficulty working and caring for her two children, ages 6 and 8. She has to call into work as sick frequently because she gets very little sleep and aches "all over". Her physician gave her a prescription-strength NSAID (ibuprofen), which has provided very little pain relief. She appears to be depressed and tells you, "I just can't cope with this pain for much longer. It is always a 6/10, if not higher. I can't work regularly. How will I support my children? Can't they give me something for this pain?"
>
> ### Questions
> **1. Does Jane have fibromyalgia? If you answer yes, what symptoms represent a possible diagnosis of fibromyalgia?**
> Aches all over, sleep disturbance, depression, fatigue.
>
> **2. What treatment would benefit Jane?**
> Amitriptyline, cyclobenzaprine, cardiovascular exercise, CBT, tramadol for pain.
>
> **3. How can you as a nurse help Jane learn to live with her condition?**
> Jane needs help coping with her daily stress and pain. Patient education about her condition and a referral to a support group can help. As a nurse caring for Jane, assuring her you believe she has pain and expressing empathy for her pain can help her feel supported. Providing positive feedback for Jane can also help improve her self image and self esteem.

Patients with a history of substance abuse

Some of the hardest patients to care for are those with a history of substance abuse who have pain. The Joint Commission states that all patients, including those with a history of substance abuse, have the right to have their pain assessed and treated (JCAHO 2000). The ASPMN has a position statement on treating pain in patients with addictive disease (ASPMN 2002). However, there is still bias and uncertainty when trying to treat these patients when they have pain.

Addictive disorders are fairly common in the United States; for example, the occurrence of alcohol abuse is 23.8% for men of all ages and 4.7% for women (Jage & Bey 2000). Substance abuse for illicit drugs is ranked at 7.7% for men and 4.8% for women (Jage & Bey 2000). Research indicates

that one in three adults who try heroin will become addicted to it (Warlitier et al 2004). Many

heroin addicts also are dependent on other drugs, such as cocaine (Jage & Bey 2000, Warltier

et al 2004).

Prescription drug abuse has grown recently: Between 1999 and 2000, there has been a 68%

increase in abuse of oxycodone and a 31% increase in abuse of hydrocodone (Warltier et al 2004).

Given the high incidence of substance abuse, it is probable that many of these patients who are

classed as addicts or who have a history of substance abuse will be seen in the healthcare system

with complaints of pain.

Difference between dependency and addiction

In order to discuss this patient population it is important to understand the correct terms for opioid

use. It is critical to understand that those patients who take opioids regularly for pain relief are not

addicts—they are classed as opioid dependent. There is a distinct difference in the two terms.

Addiction: Addiction is a chronic neurobiologic disease (APS, ASAM, APAM 2001). It is character-

ized by the four c's:

- Craving for the substance

- Compulsive use

- Lack of Control over substance use

- Continued use despite harm

Because addiction is a chronic illness and cellular changes occur with repeated substance abuse,

the potential for relapse is high (Nestler 2001). Addicts have many more mu (opioid-binding) sites on their neurons and have extra neuronal sprouts. This means that pain will be felt more easily and that the requirements for pain medication will be higher (Mitra & Sintra 2004). Many healthcare practitioners are reluctant to treat pain in addicts and patients with a history of substance abuse because they fear re-addicting the patients and drug diversion.

Opioid dependency: Patients who take opioids regularly for pain relief are not addicts; they are considered opioid dependent. This means that if they stop taking the opioid, their bodies would experience withdrawal symptoms such as nausea, vomiting, diarrhea, shaking, and elevated blood pressure. These patients are dependent on opioids for pain relief in much the same way a patient with hypertension is dependent on anti-hypertension medications to control blood pressure. Opioid dependency is not addiction. These patients are very different from the addict population, and they should not be labeled as such.

Tolerance: Tolerance is a normal physiologic consequence of continued use of a medication over a period of time. It occurs when one of the effects of the medication—sedation, nausea, or pain relief—is reduced. (Warltier et al 2004). Over time, the effect of a medication on pain relief may lessen and higher doses of pain medication may be needed to control pain. This is not a sign of addiction but of physiologic accommodation to the drug's effect over time (Jage & Bey 2000).

Opioid pseudoaddiction: Opioid pseudoaddiction is a set of behaviors that appear to indicate addiction, such as clock watching (where patients watch the clock until the next dose is due), but that are caused by undertreated pain. When patients do not get the pain medications they need to relieve pain, behaviors that are often seen as addictive, such as "drug seeking," occur. Patients are merely looking for relief but may find that by asking for pain medication each time it is due they are classed as a "clock watcher" or as "drug seeking." Once pain medication is adjusted to provide adequate pain relief, these patient behaviors resolve.

Patients with a history of substance abuse are entitled to pain relief. However, the healthcare system does not understand how to work with this patient population effectively. The physiologic changes and the psychological dependence are difficult to deal with without a multidisciplinary approach, which may require a team of a pain physician, psychologist, addictionologist, and written patient agreements that define the parameters of the care that will be provided.

Case study: Peter Shaw

Peter is a 35-year-old patient with a history of heroin use when he was in college. He now has low back pain that is interfering with his ability to work. He requires medication for his pain, and his physician is willing to prescribe an opioid medication for Peter with these parameters: Peter will sign an agreement that indicates he will receive his pain medication only from the pain clinic; the opioids will be discontinued if Peter obtains opioids from other sources; urine screening will be random and done at least twice per year, and should Peter test positive for a drug of abuse, the opioids will be discontinued. Peter is given information on the definition of addiction and opioid dependency. He is also requested to remain in contact with his sponsor in Narcotics Anonymous. Peter rates his low back pain as 7/10 and hopes that with the use of an opioid he can return to work and find some relief from his pain.

Questions

1. Once Peter starts his opioid for pain relief, will he be an addict or opioid dependent?

Peter has a history of addiction, so he will always be an addict. When he is taking medication for pain and the pain is the only reason he is taking the medication, he is considered opioid dependent. So the correct classification for Peter would be opioid dependent with a history of substance abuse.

2. Are the strict parameters of Peter's treatment plan objectionable?

Peter should expect that a healthcare provider will want to focus on the pain but at the same time protect Peter from his potential for re-addiction. By setting strict parameters for the treatment used for all patients on opioid therapy, Peter is assured of the safest care possible. The agreement also protects the healthcare provider from any accusations of providing an addict with addictive substances.

3. What other options should be considered for Peter's plan of care?

Peter should continue with his 12-step program and use non-pharmacologic methods for pain control as well. He may find that relaxation will reduce any anxiety, or that imagery may help decrease pain.

Pain management in elderly patients

Pain in older patients is often underrated and undertreated. As many as 80% of patients in long-term care facilities experience chronic pain (AGS 2002). For these patients, pain may be seen as part of aging by both the patients and the healthcare providers. Elderly patients who live in the wider community, rather than in long-term care, experience pain at lower rates—25% to 50% lower than those in nursing homes. This can be attributed to the fact that elderly people with poor health are often cared for in nursing homes (AGS 2002).

Pain medications are taken several times per week by one in five elderly patients. The low incidence of pain medication use and the high level of pain suggest a significant imbalance in treating pain in the elderly. The result of this undertreated pain in older persons can cause depression, anxiety, decreased socialization, sleep disturbances, impaired ambulation, and increased healthcare utilizations and subsequent costs (AGS 2002).

Finances are a critical part of an older patient's access to healthcare. When choosing strategies for pain relief, nurses should have a basic knowledge base on the reimbursement for medications and treatments, which will help older adults afford their medications and therapy while providing better pain relief and decreasing anxiety about affording care.

Older patients often have chronic conditions—such as diabetes, which can lead to diabetic neuropathy, or arthritis, which can become debilitating. The AGS recommends these types of treatment for older patients who have pain:

- Around the clock doses of acetaminophen with dose reductions for patients with regular alcohol use or liver impairment

- NSAID therapy for good candidates with no history of cardiac disease

- Opioids with careful titration and treatment for side effects, such as constipation

- Use of adjuvant medication, such as antidepressants or antiseizure medication, after careful consideration of all the medications a patient is taking

- Around the clock dosing is suggested for pain that is experienced over the period of the day/night, and extended-release medication when pain is present continuously

- There is no evidence to support the use of placebos

- Careful titration of all medications to avoid drug accumulation and toxicity

- Frequent reevaluation to determine whether dosing is effective and side effects are being managed adequately

(AGS 2002)

Aside from medication management for pain, the AGS recommends continued physical activity or physical therapy, patient education, and cognitive behavioral therapy that can improve self image and help with coping skills (AGS 2002). Other non-pharmacologic therapies— such as heat, cold, analgesic balms, TENS units, or acupuncture—may also be useful (AGS 2002).

By using careful assessment and prescribing, coupled with frequent reevaluation and a multimodal approach, pain can be relieved in many patients who were once thought too old to tolerate these types of therapies.

 Pain Management: Evidence-Based Tools and Techniques for Nursing Professionals

Practice exercises

1. Access the Web sites for the American Geriatrics Society, The Fibromyalgia Association, and The Chronic Pain Association, and find patient education materials that can be used to help educate patients with pain who have these pain syndromes.

2. Choose one of the case studies presented in this chapter, and develop a plan of care that addresses the specific needs of this population.

Bibliography

Agency for Health Care Policy and Research (1992). *Acute Pain Management: Operative or Medical Procedures and Trauma.* Rockville, MD: U.S. Department of Health and Human Services, Public Health Service.

Agency for Health Care Policy and Research (1992). *Clinical Practice Guideline: Acute Pain Management: Operative or Medical Procedures and Trauma.* Rockville, MD: U.S. Department of Health and Human Services, Public Health Service.

Agency for Health Care Policy and Research (1994). *Acute Low Back Problems in Adults: Assessment and Treatment.* Rockville, MD: U.S. Department of Health and Human Services, Public Health Service.

American College of Rheumatology (2000). "Recommendations for the medical management of osteoarthritis of the hip and knee." *Arthritis and Rheumatism* 42 (9): 1905–1915.

American Geriatrics Society (1998). "Clinical practice guidelines: The management of chronic pain in older persons." *Journal of the American Geriatrics Society* 46 (5), 635–651.

American Geriatrics Society (2002). "The Management of Persistent Pain in Older Persons—The American Geriatric Society Panel on Persistent Pain in Older Persons." *Journal of the American Geriatrics Society* 50 (6): 205-224.

Bibliography

American Pain Society (1997). *The Use of Opioids in the Treatment of Chronic Pain: A Consensus Statement from the American Academy of Pain Medicine and the American Pain Society.* Retrieved from *www.ampainsoc.org/advocacy/opioids.htm.*

American Pain Society (1999). *Guideline for the Management of Acute and Chronic Pain in Sickle Cell Disease.* Glenview, IL: American Pain Society.

American Pain Society (2001). "Definitions related to the use of opioids for the treatment of pain: A consensus document from the American Academy of Pain Medicine, The American Pain Society, and The American Society of Addiction Medicine." Available from *www.asam.org/pain/definitions2.pdf.*

American Pain Society (2002). *Guideline for the Management of Pain in Osteoarthritis, Rheumatoid Arthritis, and Juvenile Chronic Arthritis.* Glenview, IL: American Pain Society.

American Pain Society (2003). *Principles of Analgesic Use in the Treatment of Acute and Cancer Pain (5th ed).* Glenview, IL: American Pain Society.

American Pain Society (2005). *Guideline for the Management of Cancer Pain in Adults and Children.* Glenview, IL: American Pain Society.

American Pain Society (2005). *Fibromyalgia Pain Guideline.* Glenview, IL: American Pain Society.

American Pain Society (2006). *Pain Control in the Primary Care Setting.* Glenview, IL: American Pain Society.

American Society for Pain Management Nursing (2002). *Core Curriculum for Pain Management Nursing.* Philadelphia, PA: Saunders.

American Society for Pain Management Nursing (2002). *Position Statement: Pain Management in Patients with Addictive Disease.* Available at *www.aspmn.org/pdfs/Addictive%20Disease.pdf.*

American Society for Pain Management Nursing (2006). *Position Statement: Authorized and Unauthorized ("PCA by Proxy") Dosing of Analgesic Infusion Pumps.* Available at *www.aspmn.org/Organization/documents/PCAbyProxy-final-EW_004.pdf.*

American Society of Perianesthesia Nurses (ASPAN) (2003). "Pain and Comfort Clinical Guidelines." *Journal of Perianesthesia Nursing,* 18 (4): 232–236.

Anderson, R., Saiers, J., Abram, S., Schlicht, C. (2001). "Accuracy in equianalgesic dosing: Conversion dilemmas." *Journal of Pain and Symptom Management,* 21 (5): 397–406.

Angolara, R.T., Donato, B.J. (1991). "Inappropriate pain management results in high jury award." *Journal of Pain and Symptom Management,* 6 (7): 407.

Apfelbaumm, J., Chenm, C., Mehtam, S., Tongm, G. (2003). "Postoperative pain experience: Results from a national survey suggest postoperative pain continues to be undermanaged." *Anesthesia and Analgesia,* 97 (2): 534–540.

Arnstein P. (2002). "Theories of pain" in *Core Curriculum for Pain Management Nursing.* St. Marie, B., (ed.) Philadelphia: Saunders.

Ashburn, M., Caplan, R., Carr, D., Connis, R., Ginsberg, B., Green, C., Lema, M., Nickinovich, D., Rice, L.J. (2004). "Practice Guidelines for Acute Pain Management in the Perioperative Setting." *Anesthesiology,* 100 (6): 1–15.

Assendelft, W., Morton, S., Yu, E., Suttorp, M.J., Shekelle, P. (2006). "Spinal manipulative therapy for low back pain." *Cochrane Database of Systemic Reviews,* 2, 2006.

Australian and New Zealand College of Anaesthetists and Faculty of Pain Medicine (2005). *Acute Pain Management: Scientific Evidence.* Melbourne, Australia: Australian and New Zealand College of Anaesthetists and Faculty of Pain Medicine.

Bibliography

Ballas, S.K. (1998). *Sickle-Cell Pain*. Seattle, WA: IASP Press.

Berry, P.H. et al. (eds) (2003). *Improving the Quality of Pain Management through Measurement and Action*. Reston, VA: National Pharmaceutical Council, Inc.

Berry, P.H., Covington, E., Dahl, J., Katz, J., Miaskowski, C. (2006). *Pain: Current Understanding of Assessment, Management, and Treatments*. Reston, VA: National Pharmaceutical Council, Inc. and the Joint Commission on Accreditation of Healthcare Organizations.

Bezyack, M. (2006). "The Dangers of PCA by Proxy." *Nursing Spectrum*: 1–5.

Burkhardt, C.S. (2002). "Nonpharmcolgic management strategies in fibromyalgia." *Rheumatic Diseases Clinics of North America*, 28: 291–304.

Caldwell, J., Rapoport, R., Davis, J., Offenberg, H., Marker, H., Roth, S., Yuan, W., Sliot, L., Babul, N., Lynch, P. (2002). "Efficacy and safety of a once a day morphine formulation in chronic moderate to severe osteoarthritis pain: Results from a randomized, placebo controlled, double blind trial and an open label extension trial." *Journal of Pain and Symptom Management*. 23 (4): 278–291.

Camp, L.D., O'Sullivan, P. (1987). "Comparison of medical, surgical, and oncology patients' descriptions of pain and nurses' documentation of pain assessments." *Journal of Advanced Nursing*, 12: 593–598.

Cervero, F. (2005). "The Gate Control Theory, Then and Now" in *The Paths of Pain*. Mersky, H., Loeser, J., and Dubner, R., (eds.) Seattle WA: IASP Press.

Chevlan, E. "Opioids: A Review." *Current Pain and Headaches Report*, 7: 15–23.

Choiniere, M., Melzack, R., Girard, N., Rondeau, J., Paquin, M.J. (1989). "Comparisons between patients' and nurses' assessment of pain and medication efficacy in severe burn injuries." *Pain*, 40: 143–152.

Chok, B. (1998). "An overview of the Visual Analogue Scale and the MCGill Pain Questionnaire." *Physiotherapy Singapore*, 1 (3): 88–93.

Clarke, J.A., van Tulder, M.W., Blomberg, S.E.I., de Vet, H.C.W., van der Heijden, G.J., Bronfort, G. (2006). "Traction for low back pain." *Cochrane Database of Systemic Reviews*, 2, 2006.

Cohen, M., Smetzer, J. (2005). "Patient-controlled analgesia safety issues." *Journal of Pain and Palliative Care Pharmacotherapy*. 19 (1): 45–50.

Cole, B.H. and Brunk, Q. (1999). "Holistic interventions for acute pain episodes: An integrative review." *Journal of Holistic Nursing*, 17 (4): 384–96.

Dahl, J. and Kehlet, H. (2006). "Postoperative pain and its management." In McMahon, S.B., Koltzenburg, M. (eds.) *Wall and Melzack's Textbook of Pain*, 5th ed. Churchill Livingstone.

D'Arcy, Y.M. (1999). "A three site comparison of physician and nurse knowledge and attitudes regarding pain and patient satisfaction with pain management." Vienna, Austria: World Congress on Pain.

D'Arcy, Y.M. (2003). Chapter 2, *Pain Assessment in Medical-Legal Aspects of Pain and Suffering* (ed. P. Iyer). Tucson, AZ: Lawyers and Judges Publishing Company.

D'Arcy, Y. (2004). "Using technology to help alleviate pain." *Nursing Management*, 35 (11).

D'Arcy, Y.M. (2005). "Hot topics in pain management: NSAIDs." *Nursing 2005* 36 (2): 22–3.

D'Arcy, Y.M. and McCarberg, B. (2005). "New fibromyalgia pain management recommendations." *The Journal for Nurse Practitioners* 1 (4): 218–225.

D'Arcy, Y.M. (2005). "Conquering Pain: Have you tried these new techniques?" *Nursing 2005*, 35 (3): 36–41.

D'Arcy, Y.M. (2006). "Pain assessment and management" in *Medical Legal Aspects of Medical Records*: Tucson, AZ: Lawyers and Judges Publishing Company, Inc.

D'Arcy Y. (2006). "Treatment strategies for low back pain." *The Nurse Practitioner Journal*, 31 (4): 16–27.

D'Arcy Y. (2006). "The pain that keeps on going: Management strategies for chronic pain." *Nursing Made Incredibly Easy*, 4 (4): 37–43.

D'Arcy Y. (2007). "What's the Diagnosis?" *The American Nurse Today* 1 (4).

Daut, R.L., Cleeland, C.S., Flannery R. (1983). "Development of the Wisconsin Brief Pain Questionnaire to assess pain in cancer or other diseases." *Pain*, 17: 197–210.

Drayer, R.A., Henderson, J., Reidenberg, M. (1999). "Barriers to better pain control in hospitalized patients." *Journal of Pain and Symptom Management*, 17 (6): 434–440.

Dickenson, A. and Besson, J.M. (2005) "Pharmacological control of pain: Nonopioid targets." In Mersky, H., Loeser, J., Dubner, R. The Paths of Pain. Seattle, WA: IASP Press.

Dillard, J. and Knapp, S. (2005). "Complementary and alternative pain therapy in the emergency department." *Emergency Medical Clinics of North America*, (23): 529–549.

Donovan, M., Dillon, P., McGuire, L. (1987). "Incidence and characteristics of pain in a sample of medical, surgical inpatients." *Pain* 30: 69–78.

Dubner, R. (2005). "Plasticity in central nociceptive pathways." In *The Paths of Pain: 1975-2005*. Merskey, H., Loeser, J., Dubner, R. (eds.) Seattle, WA: IASP Press.

Dworkin, R., Backonja, M., Rowbotham, M., Allen, R., Argoff, C., Bennett, G., Bushnell, C., Farrar, J., Galer, B., Haythornthwaite, J., Hewitt, D.J., Loeser, J., Max, M., Saltarelli, M., Schmader, K., Stein, C., Thompson, D., Turk, D., Wallace, M., Watkins, L., Weinstein, S. (2003). "Advances in neuropathic pain: Diagnosis, mechanisms, and treatment recommendations." *Archives of Neurology*, 60 (11): 1524–1534.

Edwards, A. (2002). "Physiology of pain" in *Core Curriculum for Pain Management Nursing*. Saunders: Philadelphia, PA.

Feldt, K.S., Ryden, M.B., Miles, S. (1998). "Treatment of pain in cognitively impaired compared with cognitively intact older patients with hip fractures." *Journal of the American Geriatrics Society*, 46: 1079–1085.

Feldt, K.S. (2000). "The checklist of Non-verbal Pain Indicators (CNPI)." *Pain Management Nursing*, 1 (1): 13–21.

French, S.D., Cameron, M., Walker, B.F., Reggars, J.W., Esterman, A.J. (2006). "Superficial heat or cold for low back pain." *Cochrane Database for Systemic Reviews* (2), 2006.

Furlan, A.D., Brosseau, L., Imamura, M., Irvin, E. (2006). "Massage for low back pain." *Cochrane Database for Systematic Reviews* (2), 2006.

Galer, B.S. and Dworkin, R.H. (2000) *A Clinical Guide to Neuropathic Pain*. Minneapolis: McGraw-Hill.

Ger, L., Ho, S., Sun, W., Wang, M. Cleeland, C. (1999). "Validation of the Brief Pain Inventory in a Taiwanese population." *Journal of Pain and Symptom Management*, 18 (5): 316–22.

Gelinas, C., Fillion, L., Puntillo, K., Viens, C., Fortier, M. (2006). "Validation of the Critical Care Pain Observation Tool in adult patients." *American Journal of Critical Care*, 15 (4): 420–427.

Gevirtz, C. (2005). "Update on the treatment of Phantom Limb Pain." *Topics in Pain Management*, 20 (9): 1–6.

Gimbel, J.S., Richards, P., Portnoy, R. (2003). "Controlled release oxycodone for pain in diabetic neuropathy: A randomized controlled trial." *Neurology*, 60 (6): 927–934.

Ginsberg, B., Sinatra, R., Adler, L., Crews, J., Hord, A., Laurito, C., Ashburn, M. (2003). "Conversion to oral controlled release oxycodone from intravenous opioid analgesia in the postoperative setting." *Pain Medicine*, 4 (1): 31–38.

Glajchen, M. (2001). "Chronic Pain: Treatment barriers and strategies for clinical practice." *Journal of the American Board of Family Pracitioners*, 14 (3): 211–218.

Graham, C., Bond, S., Gerkovich, M., Cook, M. (1980). "Use of the McGill Pain Questionnaire in the assessment of cancer pain: Replicability and consistency." *Pain*, 8: 377–387.

Goldenberg, D.L., Burckhardt, C.S., Crofford, L. (2004). "Management of Fibromyalgia syndrome." *Journal of the American Medical Association*, 292: 2388–2395.

Gordon, D., Pellino, T., Miaskowski, C., McNeill, J.A., Paice, J., Laferriere, D., Bookbinder, M. (2002). "A 10-year review of quality improvement monitoring in pain management: Recommendations for standardized outcome measures." *Pain Management Nursing*, 3 (4): 116–130.

Grossman, S.A., Scheidler, V., Sweeden, K., Mucenski, J., Piandosi, S. (1991). "Correlation of patient and caregiver ratings of cancer pain." *Journal of Pain and Symptom Management*, 6: 53–57.

Hall, L., Oyen, L., Murray, M. (2001). "Analgesic agents: Pharmacology and application in critical care." *Critical Care Clinics*, 17 (4): 1–21.

Hagan, K.B., Hilde, G., Jamtvedt, G., Winnem, M. (2005). "Bed rest for acute low back pain and sciatica." *Cochrane Database of Systemic Reviews*, Volume 3.

Harden, N. (2005). "Pharmacotherapy of Complex Regional Pain Syndrome." *Physical Medicine and Rehabilitation*, 84 (3): S17–S28.

Harrison, A. (1991). "Assessing patients' pain: Identifying reasons for error." *Journal of Advanced Nursing* 16: 1018–1025.

Harwood, D.M., Hawton, K., Hope, T., et al. (2006). "Life problems and physical illness as a risk factor for suicide in older people: A descriptive and case control study." *Psychological Medicine*, 36 (9): 1265–1274.

Herr, K.A. and Mobily, P. (1993). "Comparison of selected pain assessment tools for use with the elderly." *Applied Nursing Research*: 6 (1): 39-46.

Herr, K. and Garand, L. (2001). "Assessment and measurement of pain in older adults." *Clinics in Geriatric Medicine*, 17 (4): 1–22.

Herr, K., Bjoro, K., Decker, S. (2006). "Tools for assessment of pain in nonverbal older adults with dementia: A state-of-the-science review." *Journal of Pain and Symptom Management*, 31 (2): 170–192.

Herr, K., Coyne, P., Key, T., Manworren, R., McCaffery, M., Merkel, S., Perlosi-Kelly, J., Wild, L. (2006). "Pain assessment in the nonverbal patient: Position statement with clinical practice recommendations." *Pain Management Nursing*, 7 (2): 44–52.

Himmelseher, S., Durieux, M. (2005). "Ketamine for perioperative pain management." *Anesthesiology*, 102 (1): 211–220.

Idelli, P.F., Grant, S., Neilsen, K., Parker, T. (2005). "Regional anesthesia in hip surgery." *Clinical Orthopedics and Related Research*, 441: 250–255.

Institute for Safe Medication Practices (2003). "Patient Controlled Analgesia: Making it Safer for Patients." Available at *www.ismp.org/profdevelopment/PCAMonograph.pdf*.

Institute for Safe Medication Practices (2005). "Medication Safety Alert—New Fentanyl warnings: more needed to protect patients." *ISMP*, 10 (16): 1–3.

Jensen, M.P. (2003). "The validity and reliability of pain measures in adults with cancer." *The Journal of Pain*, 4 (1): 2–21.

Joint Commission on Accreditation of Healthcare Organizations (2000). *Pain Assessment and Management: An Organizational Approach*. Oakbrook Terrace, IL: JCAHO.

Joint Commission on Accreditation of Healthcare Organizations (2004). "Patient controlled analgesia by proxy." *Sentinel Events Alert* issue 33. Oakbrook Terrace, IL: JCAHO.

Joint Commission on Accreditation of Healthcare Organizations (2005). "Focus on Five: Preventing patient controlled analgesia overdose." *Joint Commission Perspectives on Patient Safety*, October 2005.

Kawaguchim, M. (2001). "Percutaneous radiofrequency lesioning of sensory branches of the obdurator and femoral nerves for the treatment of hip joint pain." *Regional Anesthesia and Pain Medicine*, 26 (6): 576–81.

Khadlikar, A., Milne, S., Brosseau, L., Robinson, V., Saginur, M., Shea, B., Tugwell, P., Wells, G. (2006). "Transcutaneous electrical stimulation (TENS) for chronic low back pain." *Cochrane Database of Systemic Reviews, 2*.

Klepstad, P., Loge, J.H., Borchgrevink, P.C., Mendoza, T.R., Cleeland, C., Kaasa, S. (2002). "The Norwegian Brief Pain Inventory Questionnaire: Translation and validation in cancer pain patients." *Journal of Pain and Symptom Management*, 24 (5): 517–25.

Kumar, K. (2001). "Continuous intrathecal morphine treatment for chronic pain of non-malignant etiology: benefits and efficacy." *Surgical Neurology*, 55 (2): 86–88.

LaGanga, M.L., Monmanney, T. (2001). "Doctor found liable in suit over pain." *The Los Angeles Times*. June 15, 2001: A1, A34.

Lane, P., Kuntupis, M., MacDonald, S., McCarthy, P., Panke, J.A., Warden, V., Volicer, L. (2003). "A pain assessment tool for people with advanced Alzheimer's and other progressive dementias." *Home Healthcare Nurse*, 21 (1): 32–37.

Liu, S., Salinas, F.V. (2003). "Continuous plexus and peripheral nerve blocks for postoperative analgesia." *Anesthesia and Analgesia*, 96 (1): 263–272.

MacIntyre, D.L., Hopkins, P.M., Harris, S.R. (1995). "Evaluation of pain and functional activity in patellofemoral pain syndrome: Reliability and validity of two assessment tools." *Physiotherapy of Canada*, 47 (3): 164–170.

Marcus, D. (2000). "Treatment of nonmalignant chronic pain." *American Family Physician*, 61 (5): 1331–8, 1345–6.

Marks, R., Sachar, E. (1973). "Undertreatment of medical inpatients with narcotic analgesics." *Annals of Internal Medicine* 78: 173–181.

Marinella, M. (1997). "Meperidine-induced generalized seizures with normal renal function." *Southern Medical Journal*, 90 (5): 556–557.

Marin, R., Cyhan, T., Miklos, W. (2006). "Sleep disturbance in patients with chronic low back pain." *American Journal of Physical Medicine and Rehabilitation*, 85 (5): 430–435.

McCaffrey, M. and Beebe, A. (1968). *Pain: A Clinical Manual*. Philadelphia: Mosby.

McDonald, D.D., Weiskopf, C.S.A. (2001). "Adult patients' postoperative pain descriptions and responses to the Short Form McGill Pain Questionnaire." *Clinical Nursing Research*, 10 (4): 442–52.

McGuire, D. (1992). "Comprehensive and multidimensional assessment and measurement of pain." *Journal of Pain and Symptom Management*, 7 (5): 312–318.

Melzack, R. and Wall, P. (1965). "Pain mechanisms: A new theory." *Science*, 150 (699): 971-9.

Melzack, R. (1975). "The McGill Pain Questionnaire: Major properties and scoring methods." *Pain*, 1: 277–299.

Melzack, R. (1987). "The Short Form McGill Pain Questionnaire," *Pain*, 30: 191–197.

Mersky, H. (1979). "Classification of chronic pain: Description of chronic pain syndromes and definitions of pain terms." *Pain*, supplement 3: S217.

Moffett, J.K., Torgerson, D., Bell-Syer, S., et al. (1999). "Randomised controlled trial of exercise for low back pain: Clinical outcomes, costs, and preferences." *British Medical Journal* 319: 279–83.

Mystakidou, K., Mendoza, T., Tsilika, E., Befon, S., Parpa, G., Bellos, G., Vlahos, L., Leeland, C. (2001). "Greek Brief Pain Inventory: Validation and utility in cancer pain." *Oncology*, 60 (1): 35–42.

Mystakidou, K., Parpa E., Tsilika, E., Kalaidopoulou, O., Georgaki, S., Galanos, A., Vlahos, L. (2002). "Greek McGill Pain Questionnaire: Validation and utility in cancer patients." *Journal of Pain and Symptom Management*, 24 (4): 370–387.

National Center for Complementary and Alternative Medicine (2004). "Expanding Horizons of Health Care" *Strategic Plan 2005–2009*. Bethesda, MD: U.S. Department of Health and Human Services. National Institutes of Health.

National Comprehensive Cancer Network (2000). NCCN *Practice Guidelines for Cancer Pain*. Jenkintown, PA: National Comprehensive Cancer Network.

National Institutes of Health (1998). "Acupuncture." *NIH Consensus Statement*, 15 (5).

Nelemans, P.J., deBie, R.A., de Vet, H.C.W., Sturmans, F. (2006). "Injection therapy for low back pain." *Cochrane Database of Systemic Reviews*, 2, 2006.

Paice, J., Mahon, S.M., Faut-Callahan, M. (1991). "Factors associated with adequate pain control in hospitalized postsurgical patients diagnosed with cancer." *Cancer Nursing*, 14: 298–395.

Paice, J., Noskin, G., Vanagunas, A., Shott, S. (2005). "Efficacy and safety of scheduled dosing of opioid analgesics: A quality improvement study." *The Journal of Pain*, 6 (10): 639–643.

Pain Advocacy Community (2004). "Overview: The cost of pain." *Pain Advocacy Newsletter* 7. Available on *www.partnersagainstpain.com/painadvocacycommunity* (accessed January 12, 2007).

Page, G.G. (2005). "Surgery-induced immunosuppression and postoperative pain management." *ACCN Clinical Issues*, 16 (3): 302–309.

Pasero, C., McCaffery, M. (2001). "The undertreatment of pain." *American Journal of Nursing*, 101 (11): 62.

Pasero, C., McCaffery, M. (2002). Monitoring sedation: It's the key to preventing opioid-induced respiratory depression." *American Journal of Nursing*, 102 (2): 67–69.

Pasero, C. and McCaffery, M. (2004). "Pain Control: Comfort-function goals." *American Journal of Nursing*, 104 (9): 77–78.

Payen, J.F., et al, (2001). "Assessing pain in critically ill sedated patients by using a behavioral pain scale." *Critical Care Medicine*, 29 (12): 1–11.

Pavlov, I.P. (1927) *"Conditioned Reflexes"* in *Core Curriculum for Pain Management Nursing*. Saunders: Philadelphia, PA.

Puntillo, K.A., White, C., Morris, A.B., Perdue, S.T., Stanik-Hutt, J., Thompson, C.L., Wild, L. (2001). "Patients' perceptions and responses to procedural pain: Results from the Thunder Project II." *American Journal of Critical Care*, 10 (4): 238–251.

Purdum, A., D'Arcy, Y. (2006). *A Comparison of Two Behavioral Pain Scales in Intubated Intensive Care Unit Patients*. San Antonio, TX: American Pain Society.

Radbruch, L., Liock, G., Kiencke, P., Lindena, G., Sabatowski, R., Grond, S., Lehmann, K.A., Cleeland, C. (1999). "Validation of the German version of the Brief Pain Inventory." *Journal of Pain and Symptom Management*, 18 (3): 180–187.

Raiche, K.A., Osborne, T.L., Jensen, M.P., Cardenas, D. (2006). "The reliability and validity of pain interference measures in persons with spinal cord injury." *Journal of Pain*, 7 (3): 179–86.

Ricci, J.A. et al. (2005). "Pain exacerbation as a major source of lost productive time in US workers with arthritis." *Arthritis and Rheumatism*, 53 (5): 673–681.

Roper Starch Worldwide, Inc. (1999). *Chronic Pain in America: Roadblocks to Relief*. Available at *www.painfoundation.org/page.asp?file=Library/PainSurveys.htm*.

Rowbotham M., Kidd, B., Porreca, F. (2006). "Role of central sensitization in chronic pain: Osteoarthritis and rheumatoid arthritis compared to neuropathic pain." In *Proceedings of the 11th World Congress on Pain.* Flor, H., Kalso, E., Dostrovsky, J., (eds.) Seattle, WA: IASP Press.

Rozenberg, S., Deval, C., Rezvani, Y. et al. (1987). "Bedrest or normal activity for patients with acute low back pain: A randomized controlled trial." *Spine*, 2002: 27.

Ruetten, S., Meyer, O., Gondolias, G. (2002). "Epiduraoscopic diagnosis and treatment of epidural adhesions in chronic back pain syndromes of patients with previous surgical treatment: First results of 31 interventions." *Zeitschrift fur Orthoapdie und ihre Grenzgebiete.* Medline citation 22025828-English, 140 (2): 171–175.

Scholtz, J. and Woolf, C. (2006). "Neuropathic pain: A neurodegenerative disease." In *Proceedings of the 11th World Congress on Pain.* Flor, H., Kalso, E., Dostrovsky, J., (eds.) Seattle, WA: IASP Press.

Singelyn, F.J., Tanguy, F., Malisse, M., Joris, D. (2005). "Effects of intravenous patient controlled analgesia with morphine, continuous epidural analgesia, and continuous femoral nerve sheath block on rehabilitation after unilateral total hip arthroplasty." *Regional Anesthesia and Pain Medicine*, 30 (5): 452–457.

Staats, P.S., Argoff, C., Brewer, R., D'Arcy, Y., Gallagher, R., McCarberg, W., Reisner, L. (2004). Neuropathic Pain: Incorporating new consensus guidelines into the reality of clinical practice. *Advanced Studies in Medicine* 4 (7B): S542-582.

Stewart, W.F., Ricci, J.A., Chee, E., et al (2003). "Lost productivity time and cost due to common pain conditions in the US workforce." *JAMA*, 290: 2443–2454.

Tang, N.K., Crane, C. (2006). "Suicidality in chronic pain: A review of the prevalence, risk factors and psychological links." *Psychological Medicine* 36 (5): 575–86.

Bibliography

Tan, G., Jensen, M.P., Thornby, J.I., Shanti, B.F. (2004). "Validation of the Brief Pain Inventory for chronic non-malignant pain." *Journal of Pain and Symptom Management* 5 (2): 133–137.

Tittle, M.B., McMillan, S.C., Hagan, S. (2003). "Validating the Brief Pain Inventory for use with surgical patients with cancer." *Oncology Nursing Forum*, 30 (2): 325–330.

Van Tulder, M.W., Sholten, R.J., Koes, B.W., Deyo, R.A. (2006). "Non-steroidal anti-inflammatory drugs for low back pain." *Cochrane database of Systemic Reviews*, Volume 3.

Van Tulder, M.W., Jellema, P., van Poppel, M.N., Nachemson, A.L., Bouter, L.M. (2006). "Lumbar supports for prevention and treatment of low back pain." *Cochrane Database of Systemic Reviews*, 2, 2006.

Viscusi, E. (2005). "Emerging techniques in the management of acute pain: Epidural analgesia." *Anesthesia and Analgesia*, 101 (5S): S23–S29.

Viscusi, E., Reynolds, L., Tait, S., Melson, T., Atkinson, L. (2006). "An iontophoretic fentanyl patient-activated analgesic delivery system for postoperative pain: A double blind placebo study." *Anesthesia and Analgesia*, 102 (1): 188–194.

Watt-Watson, J. (1987). "Nurses' knowledge of pain issues: A survey." *Journal of Pain and Symptom Management*, 2 (4): 207–211.

Weissman, D.E., Joranson, D. and Hopwood, M.B. "Wisconsin physician's knowledge and attitudes about opioid analgesic regulations." *Wisconsin Medical Journal*, December: 671–675.

Weissman, D. and Haddox, J.D. (1989). "Opioid Pseudoaddiction: An Iatrogenic Syndrome." *Pain*, 36: 363–366.

Williams, V.S.L., Smith, M.Y., Fehnel, S.E. (2006). "The validity and utility of the BPI interference measures for evaluating the impact of osteoarthritis pain." *Journal of Pain and Symptom Management*, 31(1): 48–57.

Wilkie, D., Savedra, M., Holzemer, W., Tesler, M., Paul, S. (1990). "Use of the McGill Pain Questionnaire to measure pain: A meta-analysis." *Nursing Research*, 39 (1): 36–41.

Wong, D. and DiVito-Thomas, P. (2006). "The validity, reliability, and preference of the Wong Baker FACES Pain Rating Scale among Chinese, Japanese, and Thai children." Abstract available from authors at Wong on Web, available at *www.mosbysdrugconsult.com/WOW/op080.html*.

Wong, D. and Nix, K. (2004). "Use of the FACES pain rating tool with adults." Unpublished article.

Yi, M. (2001). "Doctor found reckless for not relieving pain." *San Francisco Chronicle*. June 15, 2001: A1, A18.

Nursing education instructional guide

Target audience

Directors of Education

Staff Development Specialists

Chief Nursing Officers

Directors of Nursing

Nurse Managers

VPs of Nursing

Nurse Preceptors

Staff Nurses

Statement of need

Nurses need to know the latest research and techniques so they may measure, manage, and treat pain effectively. This book teaches nurses how to accurately assess pain, the latest methods of treatment, and ways to manage pain in patients, such as non-pharmacologic pain control. The book can be used to quickly train nurses on the latest best practices for assessing and managing pain. The book gives nurses the tools they need to comply with The Joint Commission pain assessment requirements, such as different pain assessment scales for children and specialty populations.

The book provides evidence-based information and resources, allowing facilities to update pain management policies and procedures based on the latest evidence. (This activity is intended for individual use only.)

Educational objectives

Upon completion of this activity, participants should be able to

- describe the problems associated with pain management

- differentiate between acute, chronic or persistent pain, and malignant or cancer pain

- discuss the importance of using national guidelines for pain management in practice

- define the four stages of pain transmission

- identify the elements of pain assessment

- describe common barriers to pain assessment

- discuss various tools used for pain assessment

- identify pain assessment tools for specialty populations

- Review Joint Commission recommendations for choosing analgesia

- identify how to select a pain medication using the WHO analgesic ladder

- differentiate between medication types: opioids, non-opioids, and adjuvant medications for pain relief

- describe how cognitive behavioral techniques can be added to a pain management regimen

- discuss the use of non-pharmacologic therapies

- explain the safe implantation of patient controlled analgesia

- explain the key concepts of epidural analgesia

- discuss the role of regional analgesia techniques in acute pain management

- describe the use of new pain management techniques using ON-Q and IONSYS

- identify interventional therapies used to treat chronic pain

- determine appropriate treatment options for patients with difficult to treat pain syndromes

- identify barriers to pain management in older patients

Faculty

Yvonne M. D'Arcy, MS, CRNP, CNS, is the Pain and Palliative Nurse Practitioner at Suburban Hospital in Bethesda, MD. She received her master's degree from Winona State University in 1995 as a clinical nurse specialist, and received her nurse practitioner certificate at the University of Florida in Gainesville in 1999. In addition, she pursued doctoral studies at the University of Florida and the University of Maryland in Baltimore.

D'Arcy has served on the board of directors for the American Society of Pain Management Nurses and served as chair of the Clinical Practice Committee of the American Society of Pain Management Nurses. She is a member of the International Association for the Study of Pain, American Pain Society, and the American Academy of Nurse Practitioners. In 2005, she was voted Advance Practice Nurse of the Year at Suburban Hospital and received the Lambert Foundation Award.

D'Arcy lectures and presents nationally and internationally on such topics as chronic pain, difficult to treat neuropathic pain syndromes, and all aspects of acute pain management. She writes frequently on various pain management topics and has been published in several prominent journals. In 2006, she received the Gold Award for best How to Series from the American Society of Healthcare Publications Editors for "A Fieldguide to Pain Management." She is currently on the editorial boards of *Nursing 2006, The Journal for Nurse Practitioners*, and *The Pain Medicine News*. She also participated in a review of the 2000 American Pain Society Arthritis Pain Guidelines and is one of the reviewers for the American Pain Society Low Back Guideline, which is currently in development.

Accreditation/designation statement

HCPro is accredited as a provider of continuing nursing education by the American Nurses Credentialing Center Commission on Accreditation.

This educational activity for three nursing contact hours is provided by HCPro.

Disclosure statements

HCPro, Inc. has a conflict of interest policy that requires course faculty to disclose any real or apparent commercial financial affiliations related to the content of their presentations/materials. It is not assumed that these financial interests or affiliations will have an adverse impact on faculty presentations; they are simply noted here to fully inform the participants.

Yvonne M. D'Arcy has declared that she has no commercial/financial vested interest in this activity.

Instructions

In order to be eligible to receive your nursing contact hours for this activity, you are required to do the following:

1. Read the book *Pain Management: Evidence-Based Tools and Techniques for Nursing Professionals*

2. Complete the exam

3. Complete the evaluation

4. Provide your contact information on the exam and evaluation

5. Submit exam and evaluation to HCPro, Inc.

Please provide all of the information requested above and mail or fax your completed exam, program evaluation, and contact information to

Johanna Ravich

Continuing Education Coordinator

HCPro, Inc.

200 Hoods Lane

P.O. Box 1168

Marblehead, MA 01945

Fax: 781/639-0179

NOTE:

This book and associated exam are intended for individual use only. If you would like to provide this continuing education exam to other members of your nursing staff, please contact our customer service department at 877/727-1728 to place your order. The exam fee schedule is as follows:

Exam quantity	Fee
1	$0
2–25	$15 per person
26–50	$12 per person
51–100	$8 per person
101+	$5 per person

Continuing Education Exam

Name: _____

Title: _____

Facility name: _____

Address: _____

Address: _____

City: _____ State: _____ Zip: _____

Phone number: _____ Fax number: _____

E-mail: _____

Nursing license number: _____

(ANCC requires a unique identifier for each learner.)

Date completed: _____

1. *Which of the following pain definitions is the most patient-focused and useful for nurses?*

   a. Pain is whatever the person experiencing it says is occurring whenever the experiencing person says it does.

   b. Pain is an unpleasant sensory and emotional experience associated with actual or potential tissue damage, or described in terms of such damage.

   c. Pain is an unpleasant sensation that can range from mild, localized discomfort to agony.

   d. Pain is a perception, not a sensation.

2. Patients who have chronic pain

a. have pain that lasts beyond the normal healing period

b. have pain that lasts 6 weeks

c. always look like they are having pain

d. always need to take opioid medication

3. Patients who have acute pain

a. have pain that lasts beyond the normal healing time period

b. may have elevated blood pressure and increased heart rate

c. never look like they have pain

d. should ask for pain medication right away

4. When patients have neuropathic pain they describe their pain as

a. dull

b. achy

c. gnawing

d. painful tingling like pins and needles

5. You have a patient who has sickle cell disease. One of the best tools you could use to help this patient with their pain is

a. The Joint Commission pain standard

b. a disease specific guideline

c. position statement from a national organization

d. Commission on Accreditation of Rehabilitation Facilities pain standard

6. The four elements of pain transmission are

a. transduction, transmission, perception, and modulation

b. transduction, convection, perception, and modulation

c. transmission, perception, treatment, and conclusion

d. transmission, modulation, inhibition, and perception

7. A pain assessment should include which of the following factors?

a. Location, duration, description, opinion, and treatment recommendations

b. Location, intensity, duration, description, aggravating or alleviating factors, functional impairment, and a pain goal

c. Full history and physical

d. Complete lab workups

8. A common barrier to pain assessment is

a. fear of circulatory problems

b. lack of pain management options

c. lack of time to reassess pain

d. clinician's fear of addicting patients

9. You have a patient with chronic low back pain. The pain scale that would be most appropriate to use in assessing this patient's pain is the

    a. NPI/NRS

    b. FACES

    c. BPI

    d. PAINAD

10. You have a patient who is cognitively impaired with Alzheimer's disease. The pain scale you should use to assess this patient's pain is the

    a. NPI/NRS

    b. PAINAD

    c. FACES

    d. MPQ-SF

11. The Joint Commission requires that pain be assessed when medication is given and at regular intervals after the medication is administered. Recommended time frames for reassessment are after _____ for oral pain medications and after _____ for intravenous pain medications.

    a. 20 minutes, 5 minutes

    b. 45 minutes, 15 minutes

    c. 1 hour, 30 minutes

    d. 2 hours, 1 hour

12. The WHO Analgesic Ladder allows nurses to identify a correct group of pain medications by classifying medications based on

a. where the pain is occurring

b. how long the patient has been reporting pain

c. the level or type of pain the patient is reporting

d. the condition or illness causing the pain

13. Adjuvant medications

a. have an additive effect for pain relief, but do not by themselves relieve pain.

b. bind to mu agonist sites throughout the body. Once the medication is released from the systemic uptake, it binds to a specific receptor—mu—that then produces analgesia.

c. affect all types of prostaglandins.

d. affect the renal prostaglandins.

14. NSAIDs present an increased risk for heart attack and stroke

a. in all elderly patients

b. for pregnant patients

c. for patients with a history of cardiovascular disease

d. for patients who have had back surgery

15. Your surgical patient tells you she has pain at 8/10. What medication and route should you use?

    a. Tylenol, oral

    b. Fentanyl, IV

    c. Dilaudid, IM

    d. Percocet, oral

16. Your patient reports pain at a 5/10 level. Medications that are appropriate to treat that level pain include all but

    a. Vicodin

    b. Ultram

    c. Tylenol

    d. Percocet

17. Your patient has had multiple orthopedic surgeries, including a BKA amputation on her right leg two weeks ago. The operative leg has a continual painful tingling sensation and her sleep is disrupted. Her current pain regimen is Vicodin every 6 hours. She rates her pain at 7/10. What types of alternative therapies might help this patient with her pain?

    a. Relaxation while she is in physical therapy

    b. Distraction and relaxation in the evening to help sleep

    c. Acupuncture

    d. Massage

18. Therapeutic touch is a form of energy therapy that

a. involves the laying on of hands

b. does not involve actual touch

c. does not require a trained practitioner

d. involves the use of herbal supplements

19. You have a patient who is using patient controlled analgesia (PCA) for postoperative pain control. Which of the following statements is NOT part of safe PCA practice?

a. The patient must be educated on how to use the PCA.

b. The family must be educated that they are not to push the button for the patient.

c. Two nurses must check the prescription and all subsequent dose changes.

d. It is not necessary to document the amount of medication used as the pharmacy has a record of how many syringes are being used.

20. The two medications recommended for us with epidural analgesia are

a. morphine and fentanyl

b. dilaudid and sufentanil

c. hydrocodone and fentanyl

d. morphine and demerol

21. For patients with acute pain, regional analgesia techniques should

a. be used as the sole technique for pain control

b. be used as an adjunct technique for pain control

c. be used as a last resort technique for pain control

d. not be used

22. ON-Q is a local anesthetic delivery system that consists of a ball containing local anesthetic, which is attached to a catheter placed either directly on the femoral nerve, directly into a joint space such as a shoulder, or laced along a surgical incision. Once treatment is finished, how can the catheter be removed?

a. Removal is simple and patients do not need education.

b. Removal is a surgical procedure.

c. Removal can only be done by a healthcare provider.

d. Removal can be done by a patient who has received education on catheter removal or by a healthcare provider.

23. John is a chronic pain patient and takes opioids regularly for low back pain. During report, the nurse who took care of him on the previous shift says, "He doesn't look like he's in pain, but he wants his drugs right on schedule and knows what dose he should have. He doesn't look like he has too much pain to me and his CT scan is negative." Your best response would be:

a. I noticed the same thing myself. He keeps going down to the loading dock to smoke so he can't hurt that bad.

b. He looks like he's a drug-seeking patient to me.

c. Maybe he is getting tolerant to his pain medications and needs his dose increased.

d. John has chronic pain; he won't always look like he has pain. Patients can have chronic pain from tissue damage that does not show up on CT scans.

24. Patients with fibromyalgia

a. should be given opioids to treat their pain

b. do not have true pain

c. have three to five times the normal amount of substance P in their cerebrospinal fluid

d. have pain that can be treated easily

25. About 80% of elderly patient in long-term care facilities

a. get all the pain medication they need

b. experience chronic pain

c. don't think that being old means you have pain

d. seem to like the way their pain is managed

Continuing Education Evaluation

Name: _____

Title: _____

Facility name: _____

Address: _____

Address: _____

City: _____ State: _____ Zip: _____

Phone number: _____ Fax number: _____

E-mail: _____

Nursing license number: _____

(ANCC requires a unique identifier for each learner.)

Date completed: _____

1. *This activity met the learning objectives stated:*

   Strongly Agree   Agree   Disagree   Strongly Disagree

2. *Objectives were related to the overall purpose/goal of the activity:*

   Strongly Agree   Agree   Disagree   Strongly Disagree

          Pain Management: Evidence-Based Tools and Techniques for Nursing Professionals

3. *This activity was related to my continuing education needs:*

   Strongly Agree   Agree   Disagree   Strongly Disagree

4. *The exam for the activity was an accurate test of the knowledge gained:*

   Strongly Agree   Agree   Disagree   Strongly Disagree

5. *The activity avoided commercial bias or influence:*

   Strongly Agree   Agree   Disagree   Strongly Disagree

6. *This activity met my expectations:*

   Strongly Agree   Agree   Disagree   Strongly Disagree

7. *Will this activity enhance your professional practice?*

   Yes   No

8. *The format was an appropriate method for delivery of the content for this activity:*

   Strongly Agree   Agree   Disagree   Strongly Disagree

9. If you have any comments on this activity please note them here:

10. How much time did it take for you to complete this activity?

Thank you for completing this evaluation of our continuing education activity!

Return completed form to:

HCPro, Inc.
Attn: Johanna Ravich
200 Hoods Lane, Marblehead, MA 01945
Tel 877/727-1728
Fax 781/639-2982